Mouza Al Kaabi is an Emirati working mother of three. After graduating from the American University of Sharjah in 2013, she kick-started her career as a marketer, and soon after, established a small retail business through which she supports talented mothers who create beautifully handmade children's clothing and toys. The goal of her business is to support mothers in order for them to be able to support their families. Mouza Al Kaabi grew up appreciating and embracing culture and diversity, which is perceptible through her writing.

To my husband, Saeed, and my daughters Shereena, Mahra, and Alia without whom this book would have never been written.

Mouza Al Kaabi

THAT'S NOT WHAT THE BOOKS SAY!

AUSTIN MACAULEY PUBLISHERS™
LONDON • CAMBRIDGE • NEW YORK • SHARJAH

Copyright © Mouza Al Kaabi 2021

The right of Mouza Al Kaabi to be identified as author of this work has been asserted by the author in accordance with Federal Law No. (7) of UAE, Year 2002, Concerning Copyrights and Neighboring Rights.

All rights reserved. No part of this publication may be reproduced, stored in a retrieval system, or transmitted in any form or by any means; electronic, mechanical, photocopying, recording, or otherwise, without the prior permission of the publishers.

Any person who commits any unauthorized act in relation to this publication may be liable to legal prosecution and civil claims for damages.

This book is not intended as a substitute for medical advice from a qualified physician. Readers should consult their medical doctor, health adviser, or other competent professional before adopting any of the suggestions in this book or drawing inferences from them. This book is my own story with pregnancy, childbirth, and early motherhood.

The age group that matches the content of the books has been classified according to the age classification system issued by the National Media Council.

ISBN – 9789948834694 – (Paperback)
ISBN – 9789948834700 – (E-Book)

Application Number: MC-10-01-9191098
Age Classification: E

Printer Name: iPrint Global Ltd
Printer Address: Witchford, England

First Published 2021
AUSTIN MACAULEY PUBLISHERS FZE
Sharjah Publishing City
P.O Box [519201]
Sharjah, UAE
www.austinmacauley.ae
+971 655 95 202

How I bridged the gap between eastern and western wisdom to navigate my way through pregnancy, childbirth, and early motherhood.

Table of Contents

Synopsis	13
Preface	14
Do You Really Need Another Pregnancy Book?	
Chapter 1	18
Life in the United Arab Emirates	
The UAE	19
Cultural Evolution	21
The Entrepreneurial Spirit	24
Learning from My Mom	25
The Emirati Family	29
Getting Married	31
Married Life, UAE-Style	33
Chapter 2	35
Congratulations, It's Positive!	
Do You Really Want to Have a Child?	36
What I Thought Having a Child Would Be Like (And How Wrong I Was)	38
Work, Rest, and Play	42
Are We Ever Ready for Kids?	44
It's a Pug's Life: Momming a Living Creature	46
Names Matter, Whether It's a Baby or a Pet!	49

Happy Birthday to Me!	*51*
Chapter 3	**53**
Before the Birth	
Choosing the Right Clinic or Hospital	*56*
Prodded, Poked, and Scanned	*58*
Strap in for Your Hormone Roller Coaster	*60*
Miscarriage	*62*
Are You Buying Blue or Pink?	*63*
People Love to Give Advice (Even When They Don't Know What They're Talking About!)	*65*
So, What Should We Do and Who Should We Listen To?	*67*
Staying in Shape	*70*
Bye Bye Toes	*72*
Pregnancy Stages and What's Happening to You	*73*
Surprising Changes	*76*
Food, Glorious Food	*78*
Pregnancy Adventures and How Hyper I Get	*81*
Getting Bad News About Your Baby	*85*
Broken Leg While Pregnant	*89*
Strike a Pose: The Photoshoot	*94*
Let's Talk Books	*95*
Check Out Some Websites	*97*
Don't Forget the Videos	*98*
Time for Yourself or for the Baby?	*100*
Chapter 4	**103**
The Birth	
Your Hospital Bag	*106*

Going Through Labor	*107*
Being Induced	*110*
Make It Hurt Less with Pain Relief	*112*
All About Epidurals and Other Forms of Pain Relief	*114*
New Dads	*116*
You Still Have to Push After Your Baby Is Born!	*117*
The Hospital Reception	*119*
What Not to Wear	*124*
You're Still Contracting, Honey!	*125*
How Times Change	*126*
Giving Birth in the Old Days	*128*
Tradition Vs. Science	*131*
Chapter 5	**133**
You Have a Baby, Now What?	
Going Home with Your Child	*135*
The Baby Blues	*137*
Breastfeeding: Just Stick Your Baby on Your Boob	*141*
Things Are Going to Get Messy	*146*
What Color Is That?!	*150*
The Diaper Revolution	*152*
I Have No Idea What Time It Is	*154*
Baby Business School	*156*
Who's the Mom Around Here?	*158*
Will You Ever Have a Normal Life Again?	*161*
Too Much to Do	*163*
Getting a Good Night's Sleep	*164*
Bath Time	*166*

How to Mom in Public	*168*
The Perfect Mom	*170*
Having More Than One	*171*
Routines with More Than One	*175*
Getting the Right Help	*178*
Back to Work or Not	*184*
Find What Works for You	*186*
Nurseries	*188*
Traveling with Your Babies	*194*
Successful Trips	*197*
Road Trip Should Have Been a Nope Trip	*199*
Good Places to Visit with Kids	*201*
How to Pick a Hotel	*204*
Planes, Trains, and Automobiles	*205*
Keep Them Busy	*207*
Would They Eat the Food?	*208*
Technology	*209*

Synopsis

When I was expecting my first child, I read everything I could get my hands on about pregnancy and childbirth. My loved ones gave me volumes of advice as well, which often ran counter to what the books said and what I had come to believe from a lifetime of living in the UAE. Instead of making me feel empowered and capable, the advice left me feeling ashamed, confused, scared, incapable, and really, really down. I found myself constantly responding to people's recommendations by saying (and sometimes yelling) "THAT'S NOT WHAT THE BOOKS SAY!" – hence, the title of the book.

This book is meant to give you an insight on how you should use your own intelligence to apply the advice that works for your own lifestyle and say "no thanks" to the well-intentioned advice that doesn't; whether it comes from books, strangers, or loved ones. Because when it comes to parenting, love and happiness flow most freely when you follow your heart.

Preface
Do You Really Need Another Pregnancy Book?

Clearly, I think the answer is yes or you would not be reading this. One day, when I was tidying away my pregnancy books, I noticed something. It stopped me in my tracks and I started to take the idea of writing a book seriously.

Each book had a similar picture on the cover: a beautiful woman with either a perfect bump or a cherubic baby in her arms. However, they did not look like my daughter or myself. Not one of them.

I tipped the box out, which Shereena, my firstborn, thought was a great game, and sorted them into piles according to where the author was from. Turns out just about all of my treasured stash of pregnancy books came from the United States, some were from the U.K., and one or two came from Australia. There was not even one from an Arab country.

Whether you grew up in Sharjah, Shanghai, Sydney, or San Francisco, the mechanics of having a baby is the same for us all. Am I right? You get pregnant, your belly grows (and grows and grows), and then a new person comes out. Yet, culture is a big part of a person's identity. It colors our lives from childhood to old age, and it is an essential part of the experience of becoming a parent. Culture is ingrained in our decisions about names for our children, in our choices about what kind of care or intervention we want or have available during pregnancy and birth, and in everything we choose to do to our bodies or put in them. Nonetheless, in all the books I read, the part talking about my culture was missing, which is why after I gave birth, I found people constantly telling me to do things that did not match what I had just learned. I was constantly responding to their recommendations by saying (and sometimes yelling) *"**THAT'S NOT WHAT THE BOOKS SAY!**"*

As you read this book, you will discover my obsession with Friends, the T.V. series, and how it became a big part of my first pregnancy. I was a fan of the show from a very young age, but when I got pregnant, I found myself watching the episodes where Carol, Phoebe, and Rachel are pregnant over and over again. Nevertheless, aside from the obvious issues with a growing bump, Phoebe's experience or even Rachel's pregnancy stories were never going to be like my stories. There is something disempowering about not seeing our faces or experiences reflected by what we see on TV, film, and the Internet. If we do not see ourselves in the media around us, especially in the pregnancy and parenting advice books we read, how are we supposed to feel about that?

The Internet—with all its amazing YouTubers, the explosion of social media influencers, and sometimes the local media coming out of UAE, especially—has made things a lot better. But social media can't give us the tools and resources we need to survive, thrive, and navigate life's challenges specific to our everyday realities. People often follow advice they find on social media, even when the person posting this advice has no credentials to back up the idea they're presenting. It is a whole other side to "fake news," where often, people make things up or don't check their facts before presenting advice. We should not just take any advice because it is well designed into an Instagram post, or presented through a well-edited YouTube video. Have you noticed how normal it has become to simply skim over cultural references that do not apply to the reality of life here? It is the same on many of the websites, blogs, and books we read. And it's not just pregnancy books, but also beauty, fashion, films, and more, which often do not quite connect to life in the Arab world, especially in culturally conservative societies like the UAE.

Somehow, when it comes to motherhood-related books, our culture is not addressed at all, leaving millions of women in the dark feeling scared and alone. Women everywhere, not just in the Western world, need to know that the advice they are getting about their bump and their baby is right for them and their lifestyle. Let us face it: when it is 50 degrees outside, a dainty little sunshade is not going to help you give your infant tummy time in the park, no matter what your parenting guide says. You would be committing child endangerment. The UAE healthcare systems are vastly different from those in the UK and US, so entire chapters of the existing books are irrelevant to us, leaving us rudderless in a sea of new information.

Later that day, as I wiped down the tray of my daughter's high chair I looked at her happy, mush-covered face and realized it was well past bath time, but more importantly, I realized I should make this book happen, not just for me or for the community, but for her. I decided there was no way I was going to let my daughter grow up thinking her experiences were any less valid than those of some American comedian or British actress. Not that their experiences are completely irrelevant, but cultural differences do play a huge role in how we tackle universal experiences.

At that moment, I knew that someone should write a book about Emirati women and their experience of pregnancy and parenting, and I realized that person should be me! I knew that there were other women like me who wanted a book they could read and relate to with anecdotes and specific local views about pregnancy and childbirth here in the UAE. My mission became to create the book I wished I had when I was expecting. Until I wrote it, there was a good chance my daughter would grow up to have the same experience as me, feeling invisible in the world of pregnancy and parenting books.

Therefore, I resolved to take up the challenge to write not a parenting book for Emirati women, but some sort of a "motherhood memoir" that we all can relate to. One that would be full of relevant insights and experiences that could help a new mom in Dubai, a first-time parent in Abu Dhabi, or someone thinking about starting a family in Sharjah. I became passionate about bringing the Emirati woman's experience out of the closet and into the open so that you, dear reader, can sigh in relief as you recognize your experiences, worries, and conundrums as perfectly normal. I want my book to speak to pregnant mothers in the Emirates especially because we are torn between what is written in books that were not written anywhere close to our country and what our society believes in. I want you to know that everything will be okay; someone else has been through this whole confusion and has put her story in writing to make you feel less worried about what is coming your way.

I want to share my stories to inspire, not to tell you that this is what you have to do. If there is one takeaway you get from this book, it is this: everyone can give you "advice," but you are the only one who knows what works best for your lifestyle.

So here it is. With God's blessing, I hope you find it useful.

Chapter 1
Life in the United Arab Emirates

Learning to walk or to talk, graduating from school or university—these are some of the achievements we all strive for. As we get older, most of us marry and have children. Each of these events is like a trophy on the wall of life and can feel like a real accomplishment. But even though these milestones are really important and feel unique to us, these experiences are universal. Across the world and across cultures, people reach these pinnacles and achieve these ambitions. It is humbling to step back sometimes and recognize how these important personal events connect us to all people across the globe.

But that doesn't mean our experiences are all the same. All those parenting books I read aimed at Western women helped me see that celebrating these milestones and our experiences of them is universal but also unique to each culture, and we should embrace that. This lighthearted look at being a woman and becoming a mom in the UAE is based on my experiences and observations of life as I crossed the threshold into parenthood. I hope you enjoy this glimpse into my life and, if you are a UAE mom too, I hope it brings you relief as you learn you are completely normal and you are most definitely not alone!

In case you are not an Emirati and you are curious about the region, I would first like to fill you in on what Emirati life is like; how families do things here in the United Arab Emirates, especially my family. Feel free to skip ahead to the parenting sections if this bit is not for you. Otherwise, enjoy a peek into my culture and my country.

The UAE

"A nation without a past is a nation without a present or a future. Thanks to God, our nation has a flourishing civilization, deep-rooted in this land for many centuries. These roots will always flourish and bloom in the glorious present of our nation and in its anticipated future." –The late Shaikh Zayed Bin Sultan Al Nahyan, the founding father of the United Arab Emirates.

The United Arab Emirates is a young country. It was only founded in 1971. The new nation brought together six Emirates, with a seventh joining a year later. (Emirates are similar to kingdoms, but headed by a sheikh. We can think of sheikhs as princes.) The most famous Emirates are Dubai and Abu Dhabi. When I first moved to Abu Dhabi and then started to travel on holidays, people did not know what Abu Dhabi was when I told them where I was from. This was around 2013 and 2014. Therefore, to save myself the long conversations, I started saying that I was from Dubai. What shocked me is that in more recent years, when I tell people abroad that I am from Dubai, they tell me that they have only been to Abu Dhabi! I have also come across many people who think that Dubai is the country and Abu Dhabi is its capital. Besides Dubai and Abu Dhabi, there are also Sharjah, Ajman, Umm Al Quwain, Fujairah, and Ras al Khaimah.

The oil industry boom in the 1950s and 1960s created a lot of wealth in the Middle East. It completely underpins the extraordinary growth of Dubai and other major cities in the country, but these days we are starting to look beyond oil. Young Emiratis growing up as the cities grew have never known any other way of life. However, our grandparents and even our parents remember how the country used to be. While there were always some cities and towns on the coast, large numbers of UAE families were nomadic. There is still a romance for the old desert traditions, especially among the men in the families who sometimes drive out into the desert to camp and have fun.

Cultural Evolution

"Future generations will be living in a world that is very different from that to which we are accustomed. It is essential that we prepare ourselves and our children for that new world." –The late Shaikh Zayed Bin Sultan Al Nahyan, the founding father of the United Arab Emirates.

As a child, I believe most of us only think of the next step. We never think of five or ten years in the future until we get to that first job interview and get asked "where do you see yourself in five years?" When I was in grade three, I was excited to go to grade four. I did not have far-flung hopes of university or even high school. However, as adults, we make plans for our children's futures. We dream about who they might become and what they will do, and gradually our children learn what we dream for them. I grew up knowing that my parents always wished for me to earn a college degree. Then I would get a good job. This has been the guiding path I have followed through my life.

In the past, before the Emirates discovered oil, parents' goals for their kids were the same as they had been for generations, ever since our people first lived in this region. Moms and dads simply wanted their children to have a family and to prosper. For my culture, traditionally, having a family offers a sense of security and this is very important. Since the time of my ancestors, when the young people were ready, they got married and lived a good life raising their children. Now, however, society is changing. For my generation, for me and my sisters, living in the new skyscraping cities built on the oil wealth of our young nation, our parents' first goal for all of us was to get educated. I always knew that if marriage came, my family would be happy, it would be fine, but the big difference from the past is that if marriage did not come, that would also be okay. It is not the main thing for us anymore, and that is true for both boys and girls.

This interest that came from what I would assume the 1980s onwards in higher education for both men and women has been a real cultural shift from the past for Emirati families, but it's been very positive and very gradual. What I love is that our roots in the values that make Emirati families strong are still as solid as ever, and our lifestyles continue to revolve around family gatherings and events. But we live in a world that appears on the surface to be incredibly modern; it embraces new technology and is full of ambition. As a nation, we are using our oil wealth, our innovative plans, and many other achievements that are not centered around oil anymore to be very outward and forward-looking. We live and work digitally, we welcome visitors from across the world to work among us, and all of this gives us a global view and a thirst for travel.

I am Emirati through and through: I was born in Dubai in 1990, raised in Sharjah, and now reside in Abu Dhabi with my husband Saeed and three children, Shereena, Mahra, and Alia. However, like so many young Emiratis, I was educated in American institutes. I grew up speaking both English and Arabic. What has contributed a lot to my English was that my brother married an American who moved in my family's house in 1999—my American sister who lived with us for a period of time. I grew up watching Disney classics in English, and series like "Sabrina the Teenage Witch" and "Clueless." I still watch English and American movies and TV shows on daily basis, and my all-time favorite show is "Friends." I would reference each and every situation that happens in my life to a joke said on the show or a situation that happened to the characters of the show. My peers and I have grown up in a time and place that sits right in the middle of two wealthy cultures, and that gives us a unique perspective on them both. I enjoy much about Western media and culture, but I respect our Emirati traditions as well, and I apply them both with logic. This is a typical modern way of life for young people here in UAE, and it is one reason why I see our nation as a real crossroads of the world.

The Entrepreneurial Spirit

In my experience, Emirati women have always had an entrepreneurial spirit. However, that spirit has not always been something that could be encouraged or accommodated because of the importance of bearing many children. Women in the past used to work on what is now referred to as "traditional crafts." They used to make *khous*, which are handwoven palm leaves traditionally used for roofing and floor mats, or *telli*, the most cherished form of embroidery in the UAE, or *sadu*, which is handwoven wool traditionally used in making Bedouin tents and carpets. Henna art, sewing, and pottery were also part of a traditional craft repertoire. Looking back at my mother's and grandmother's generations, women in our family married young, the minute they were ready to have children. They were proud to have many children for the family and raised them with very little help. Their lives were full of love but also full of hard work like house chores, sometimes cooking feasts for the entire neighborhood, as such generosity is embedded within the culture. Often, women managed all this and created businesses too. My mother is a fantastic example of an entrepreneurial Emirati woman. She built up a clothes-making business and has been an inspiration for me as I explore my options as a woman, a mother, and a budding entrepreneur as well.

Learning from My Mom

I grew up in Sharjah, and when I was a little girl, I was surrounded by the most fantastic fashion. Design and fashion grew to be a passion of mine, and I am sure this is all because of my mother. Besides having eight children, my talented mother created her own fashion empire—or at least to my 6-year-old self it was an empire. Back when I was small, we did not have all the malls and international fashion stores that the UAE is famous for today. Instead, many clothes were handmade and designed locally. My mother saw there was a market for beautiful dresses, skirts, and with exquisitely detailed embroidery, so she set up her own designer tailor shop. Clients would come in and she would create pieces especially for them: bespoke, made-to-measure. She had a large team of seamstresses and tailors to custom-make her designs, and the clients loved her work. They told other people about her, and hers became one of the most successful tailoring shops in Sharjah between 1996 and 2000.

I used to go to Mom's shop from the age of six to watch her work. It was magical being there surrounded by this creative team and all the rolls of colorful fabric, seeing the machines at work and the skills of the craftspeople as they sewed the fine detail. But behind it all was the talent of my mother. Her friends love to remind me of the times when they visited the shop when I was little and I pretended to be the designer, sketching out designs for them and wasting a ton of my mother's paper! I am sure this is where my own love for design and fashion comes from. When I went to high school, a dream grew inside me that after getting a sensible degree in business or some other "substantial" subject, I would pursue a degree in fashion as well. Then I would follow my mother's footsteps.

Nevertheless, my mother's fashion dream did not last long. She became a victim of her own success and the jealousy of others. Local designers saw what was happening and were envious of her growing client list. People started bribing her tailors and taking them away to open their own businesses. Running the shop became so much harder than simply designing beautiful clothes for people. In the end, it became too stressful and, when I was ten, she sold the business.

I still love fashion and I have inherited my mother's entrepreneurial spirit. At university, I got my first chance to test this out. In 2008, I set up a successful fashion blog called *Fashion Hermit*. It was all about having a different style from everyone else. I wrote about the recent trends, and people started to follow my blog. Back then, setting up a blog was somewhat new; only a few Emirati girls were doing it. The idea of being a fashion designer was too far out there. People did not see it as a real career option. But that blog gave me an amazing opportunity when I was offered the chance to work as a fashion editor for an online Dubai magazine called *Style in Dubai*.

I would go to the shops, have photoshoots, and get invited to exclusive events. I met designers such as Tom Ford, Michael La Coste, and Antonio Marras. It was such a fun time and really exciting for me. But when I got engaged and was almost done with university, it felt like it was the right time to end that chapter. It's important to do what suits your life and let things go when they don't work for you anymore.

I no longer see myself working in fashion, but I still take pride in my appearance and I enjoy fashion on a personal level. I love dressing myself, I love helping my sisters and friends make the right fashion choices when they ask me for help. What is interesting, though, is that now a lot of local designers have emerged, achieving successes on an international scale, especially since 2013. We are seeing an exciting boom in local talent and creativity, which is excellent for the country. There are hundreds of Emirati labels to choose from now. But I love how my mother was a trailblazer and, through my blog, in a way so was I. I recently met someone who had also gone to school in Sharjah, and we were surprised to find out that we were neighbors who had never met. She went home and spoke about me to her sister who responded by saying, "Mouza Al Kaabi? From Sharjah? Got married and moved to Abu Dhabi? She was the first Emirati blogger!" I modestly admitted that was me, but surely I was not the first Emirati blogger.

So I had this hope of working in fashion and, for as long as I can remember, I wanted to visit Paris, the fashion capital of the world. I finally took a trip there at the age of twenty (2010), and it was everything I had hoped it would be. I really loved the city. Moreover, I remember walking with my sister's friend and telling her, "Mark my words, someday I'm going to live here and I'm going to set up my own label." It seemed so clear to me. But everyone's interests change over time. Especially when you are a university or a high school student, you have different interests than when you graduate and go into the workforce and see what the real world is like.

Now, I have my marketing job at a media-specialized company, a sector I strongly believe in. My current job is my second job since graduating university in 2013. At the end of 2016, I started setting up a small business selling children's clothing and toys handmade by mothers from different parts of the world. The mission of my business, Tony & Natty, is to support mothers with sewing skills in order for them to be able to support their own families. The store was launched in 2017, which was marked as "The Year of Giving" in the United Arab Emirates, and I love how my concept fit the theme of the year.

I have noticed that Emirati women seem to be different from women in many Western societies because we are juggling so many things. For my mom, it was tailoring besides raising her children. For myself and besides being a mother, I work 9 to 5 in marketing, I am writing this book, and I have my small retail business. I see opportunities all the time, and many of the women I know have a similar lifestyle. They work in an office as well as having a family, and lots of them have a little business of some kind. This seems to be a real strength of Emirati women that not every culture has.

The Emirati Family

The United Arab Emirates is at a crossroads in time and history, and you can really see that in how young couples are living these days. Our people come from a proud tradition of families who travelled the region and lived at peace with the desert landscape. In the mid-twentieth century, our nation was blessed to discover great natural riches under our desert. The skyscraping cities of Dubai, Abu Dhabi, and other Emirates have raced upwards on the wealth those discoveries created, and our families live in ways our forefathers of only a few generations ago could never have dreamed. However, despite all the changes on the surface, our traditional culture and family ways shine through, for which we are blessed.

If you are Emirati, I will bet you met your husband in the same way I met mine. Saeed and I were childhood sweethearts. The tradition here in the UAE and in the Gulf countries in general is that the parents chat together and when their friends have children, they always say, "Oh, this girl is my son's future wife" or "This is my daughter's future husband." Maybe people in other countries do something similar when their children are small. If you're a "Friends" fan, remember that episode right after Rachel gives birth to Emma when Janice walks in the hospital room with her newborn son saying, "Say hello to Aaron, your future son-in-law!"? Our situation is almost the same. It is a compliment to your friend's child saying you think they are good enough for your child to marry. And it's super cute to look at your babies and imagine their future like that, especially when they're toddling along hand-in-hand. Even in my generation, we still do it. When my friend had a son recently, I found myself saying, "Oh, that's my future son-in-law."

In Western countries, it seems that the tradition stops there when the boys and girls are babies. But here in the UAE, quite often those visions we dream of when our children are small turn out to be true, and those cute toddlers do grow up to marry each other. And before anybody starts to get concerned, no one is coerced. It is not like that. There is no pressure and it is not a rule. I have people in my family who were supposed to marry a particular person the parents wished them to marry, but it did not happen that way in the end. It is a real choice for our young people. What Western people often do not realize, though, is that in reality the parents' suggestion often works out well. We spend so much time socializing with our families, if we are able to find someone suitable from friends' families, it means we spend more time with the people we like and love. It brings people together in a lovely way.

For Saeed and I, this tradition worked out beautifully. We were childhood friends. When we were small, we used to play together, and our families used to hang out a lot with each other. Sadly, as can happen, our families grew apart for a while, so I did not see Saeed from the age of six to around sixteen or seventeen. Then I saw him again. It was just a brief "Hi, how are you? How are you doing?" and so on, but I could not stop thinking about him! Little did I know that I was on his mind, too. We were thinking about each other the whole time from that point, but our lives went in separate ways again, and we didn't speak for another five years.

Eventually, it happened that we reconnected during my last year of university, in 2011. This is quite a popular time for women to think about getting married, just as they finish their education. So, here is a fairytale for the digital age, as Rachel would say: Saeed approached me on Twitter. We realized how much we liked each other, so we decided to get married. The modern Emirati way.

Getting Married

One way our marriage culture has changed across the generations is that after the wedding we now go away on honeymoon, while in my mother's generation that barely ever happened. Saeed and I went off and enjoyed a very tranquil honeymoon in the Maldives. But when we returned from our travels, we started our married life in the traditional Emirati way, not in a home of our own, as we would do if we were English or American perhaps; instead, we came back from our travels and moved into Saeed's family's house in Abu Dhabi.

Living all together like this with the husband's family is the Emirati way. It is important for us to live together with our family members across all the generations. This is quite unlike the Western countries, where the new couple goes off and sets up a home on their own. For us, the wife moves in with her husband's family, and often this will mean living with his parents, grandparents, brothers, and unmarried sisters. Our houses usually have separate apartments inside them, so they do not feel crowded.

For me, I felt very blessed to move into Saeed's family house, as Saeed's younger sister is a talented interior designer. When we returned from our travels, we found she had lovingly prepared an apartment for us. To begin with, we shared our home with his mother, grandmother, sister, and younger brother, but his father mostly stayed in another home of theirs in Al Ain, a city in Abu Dhabi that is almost two hours away from downtown Island, due to his work. It is a sociable setup, but within the family home everyone has his or her own space. It is a lovely way to live. On the day we arrived back from our honeymoon, it was a joy to walk in and see our rooms beautifully decorated and furnished and to feel so welcomed.

Married Life, UAE-Style

When I first moved to Abu Dhabi, I did not work for six months. I had so much to get used to in this new city and I was a new wife. I developed a lovely routine at first. My husband would go to work and I would go to the gym, then pop to the salon before going grocery shopping. Sometimes, I would skip the grocery store and stay at the salon for hours, getting the most complicated nail art done! I would then head home, cook something light or order takeout for lunch, and that would be my day until he came in from work.

After six months, though, I found a job. It turned out, it was boring not working, and I felt it the most when I was on maternity leave in 2014, 8 months after getting my first job and 14 months after getting married. I was ready to go back to the office! I started working as a marketer at a government entity that does quality infrastructure for Abu Dhabi. They do all the testing to ensure that all the products and services are according to the international standards. It was a good place to start my career. In early 2018, I moved to a different sector, which is media, but still as a marketer. This type of career away from home is very different from my mom's experience and definitely a big change from what my grandmother's lifestyle was like. They were married so much younger than me and started having children much younger as well. The opportunity was not there to get a degree in the way it is now, and they didn't have the options we have. However, the founding father of the United Arab Emirates, Sheikh Zayed Bin Sultan Al Nahyan, has changed the mindset of the society and given women the right to work and be productive outside of the house. In one of his speeches he said, "The woman is half of the society; any country which pursues development should not leave her in poverty or illiteracy." The United Arab Emirates was the first Arab country to introduce a mandatory female presence in boardrooms.

Chapter 2
Congratulations, It's Positive!

I do not think anyone ever forgets the moment they learn they are pregnant for the first time. Who was there when you found out? Did you wee wee on a stick in your bathroom, or do a test in the doctor's office? Who did you tell first? Did your mom cry when she heard? Did your heart skip a beat and were you, maybe, a tiny bit scared of the seriousness of what it all meant, or were you purely excited? Suddenly, in the blink of an eye, that test result means you will become a mother and you have a new title to add to wife, daughter, and employee. Congratulations, Mommy!

Do You Really Want to Have a Child?

This question has many different answers. I sometimes wonder what I would say if I could go back in time and talk to my younger self, the one still at university maybe and the one who is still deciding what she wants to do with her life. Do not get me wrong: I am definitely still learning in life, but I already know there are so many things you cannot truly understand until you experience them. People can give you advice until they are blue in the face, but until you have lived it, you probably will not really truly understand it. This is the way of the world. However, think about it for a moment; I am sure you would have something to say if you could go back in time and talk to your younger self. Well, this is what I would say to the twenty-three-year-old Mouza fresh out of university.

First, I would just take that young woman and shake her by the shoulders! Really, I would. So many young women are far too quick to want babies, but they do not understand how life changes when a baby becomes part of the equation. Women have become used to having a lot of personal freedom. Young women in the UAE come and go almost as they please. They go shopping, meet their friends, go to the gym, and have a good job. It is wonderful and I am happy about how life is evolving here. But chuck a baby in the mix and everything changes. All that freedom starts to fade away.

Now stop. I see you there smiling to yourself. You think you will be different; you are thinking to yourself that you will just bring the baby along to dinner; you will pop the baby in a stroller and still go to the mall with your friends. Why should anything change? It is just a baby. Right? Wrong. So, so wrong. A baby changes your life like nothing else. Not even marriage comes close. That little creature becomes your new boss!

What I Thought Having a Child Would Be Like (And How Wrong I Was)

Before I got pregnant, I did not give it too much thought. Who does, really? Until you, your sisters, or your friends start having families, it is not something that's relevant. Having children is the most natural thing in the world, so I assumed it was going to be easy.

One thing I knew was how other people's children should behave. I definitely had views about other people's children. If I hung out with people with kids, or if I was at the mall and I saw people there with children and they were screaming, I used to roll my eyes. Why did they bring them? Couldn't they just make them stop? Why not leave the child at home while you do your shopping? You don't need to drag your child everywhere you go. And I wish they would just stop making so much noise! Sound familiar?

I genuinely thought I would be one of those mythical moms who would never let the children ever ruin their lives or control them. Of course, I thought, I am the mom, so I'm going to control the baby. The baby cannot control me. I will be in charge. How can someone so small be hard to manage? I believed it would be easy for me to do things with kids, not only with one kid, but also with two. I would go to the mall without them if I wanted to shop with my friends. Or I would simply put them in the stroller and look at all the clothes I wanted. I would even try things on or have lunch whenever it suited me. Oh, how I laugh at myself now. Truly, there are some things we can only learn through experience, but I hope you can learn from my mistakes, and save yourself some of the hassle I went through!

Think about it like this: before you have children, you can think your life is difficult and complicated, but really, you are free in a way you never will be again. You can come and go as you please with no one's needs to think about, except your own. Think about the act of leaving your house. It is not something you need to think about, is it? You decide you want to go out and you go out. Simple. Without a baby, you can stand up and walk out the door just because you want to. It is so straightforward and easy, and I am so envious! I am reminiscing about those easy days. You think, I want to go out, so you put on your shoes, grab your bag, and inside thirty seconds you are walking to your car. Oh, the bliss of a life like that!

But that changes when you bring a new life into the world. Going out has to be timed around feeding the baby, the baby's naps, the baby's activities, the baby's need to poop, or even the baby's mood. You need to bring a ton of equipment with you rather than just your purse. There is the stroller, the diaper bag, the toys, the changes of clothes, maybe some bottles, hot water, formula powder or food, and wipes. The list goes on. Then, just when you have got everything ready to go and finally put on your own shoes, the baby fills the diaper. By the time you've changed them they need to be fed. An hour and a half later, you give up.

But even if you do go out, you have to take your child with you everywhere you go if you didn't have any help or if you had some trust issues like I did when I first had children. At least with the first one. It's not until you first hold that new little person your body has spent the last forty weeks making that you learn an irreversible truth: you just switched positions in your own life. You are no longer the center of it. This new little person is, and sometimes you will literally sit there and watch them breathe while they sleep. They are so amazing and so important that everything else comes second for a while. After having Shereena, I found out just how hard it is to leave your child, even if you have a nanny. Sometimes the reason that a woman is out with her screaming baby is that she is really worried that something might go wrong at home because she is not there. You want to have your kids with you all the time, even when you have someone else to look after them while you run an errand!

The funny thing is that no matter what I say, you will not quite believe me. You think you can do it differently. You will be the mom who takes her child to the new shop in the mall or out for dinner; you will be different from the rest of us and your life will not change. Go ahead and keep that dream. But I can say with my hand on my heart that life before and after children is a very different thing, and not just because of practicalities like getting out the door on time. It is different for one main reason: your priorities change.

Going to that dinner party or staying late at work to get your promotion becomes less important than giving your child what they need. This is because you love them from the bottom of your soul. It is an amazing and beautiful thing and there is nothing like it. If you are already pregnant and my story has freaked you out, do not worry. It is completely and utterly worth it. The love you have for your child powers you through staying up with them to soothe them until the crack of dawn. And you'll do that whether or not you went to that party or stayed up working all night. As you hold your child and feel their warm little head start to calm and rest against your shoulder, you might start to care less about the mall and the promotion. Instead, you start valuing your own rest more because you have to cope with the new lifestyle. And you have to cope because this little person utterly needs you. You start to turn down those invitations, even if you long for the days when you were in and out freely, and you leave your computer at the office, even if you miss the days when you worked without feeling guilty. Instead, you watch your child breathe softly in their crib. And you are perfectly happy because life before children and life after children will always be in a battle in your head.

Come back and read this again after your baby is here, and everything I have said here will ring true. When it is the right time for you to become a mom, making those changes to your life will be completely worth it and you will be happy to make them. So make sure it is the right time, as you cannot send them back after they arrive! And your life of work, shopping, and parties will never be the same again.

Work, Rest, and Play

As a modern Emirati woman, I started the job hunt right after graduation and finally got a job six months after getting married and moving to Abu Dhabi. Having a career is important to me, and I always knew I would continue working after having children. I had no idea what kind of impact they would have on my daily life, though! But with modern ways, Emirati women can enjoy both a family and a career. As the world changes, it is important for girls to see good role models showing them how it can be done and how to balance all the roles we have in life. Looking back, we can see how much the world has changed since our grandparents were young. Who can imagine how different life will be fifty years from now?

But when I'm not working, I love curling up on my sofa, reading a book, on my phone, or watching some series. Another thing I enjoy adding to my schedule when time permits is going to the gym. In fact, I reached my highest level of fitness right before my first pregnancy. Going to the gym with the trainer I hired when I first moved to Abu Dhabi has always been a great way to reduce stress and I loved the way it made me feel. Sadly, though, my favorite trainer had to move back to her country after training me for three years, and just like that, gym has not been fun anymore.

The main way, however, that my husband and I enjoy ourselves is to socialize with our friends and family. Visiting friends and family is such a big part of our culture and I love it. We would drive to my family in Sharjah and his family in Al Ain or catch up with friends at a newly opened cafe or restaurant in Dubai, which often feels like a weekly event. I think this is one of the strongest parts of Emirati society. It is not something we only do during Eid or special occasions; it is a big part of our daily lives. And while some things are different, that didn't change when our children arrived.

Are We Ever Ready for Kids?

Before we started our own family, I did not have much experience with children. Although I am an aunt to a number of nieces and nephews, I had never really taken care of a baby before. Thinking back, I do not think I was actually that fond of children. I might have played with them for a few minutes when they were being quiet and well behaved. But always with their mothers around! I was never left in charge of any of them and I certainly never had to deal with a screaming baby or change a poopy diaper!

When we were first married, I always felt as though there was a lot of time ahead of us. We were in no rush. Especially as having a baby means immense responsibility. I could see that in how my sisters and friends had to manage their children. They could not just sit and chat freely with me anymore. Our socializing definitely changed with them after they had children. In addition, I did not think I was ready for that at the beginning of my marriage! But five months into it, the topic of babies had come up a lot of times. Saeed and I started playing with our nieces and nephews in a fonder manner and I started thinking it might be a good plan. I started noticing more of the cute baby things you could get when you had children, and the idea grew on me.

On one of our trips to the mall, Saeed and I were at one of the department stores and I saw a Dior baby bottle. I found these utterly adorable. I mentioned to Saeed how I had always loved seeing my sisters use them for their children. So, my husband said I should get one. But as soon as he said this, I started to have doubts. Could buying a baby bottle when we were not yet expecting be bad luck? What if I had some kind of health condition that prevented me from having children?

If that were true, then the bottle would be a painful reminder of what I could never have. It would break my heart. I explained this all to my husband, but he laughed at my fantasies and insisted we buy it anyway. I gave in and we walked out with the last one in the store. It was blue. As soon as we got outside, my fears grew again. What would happen if we never had children? What if I was infertile? We had our first fight right there and then over a baby bottle for a boy we did not have. Little did I know I was already carrying an adorable little baby in my womb at that moment!

It's a Pug's Life: Momming a Living Creature

When is a dog like a baby? When you have to look after it! Pets are not for everyone, but if you are thinking about having a baby, it wouldn't hurt to see how good you are at looking after a pet first. When you have an animal in your home, it is your job to keep the darn cute thing alive but also to deal with all the icky bits and medical stuff. Pets are definitely less demanding than human babies, which makes pet ownership a good stepping stone.

When I was a little girl, I pleaded and pleaded to have a pet until my parents caved in. I was so excited when they finally said yes, but my joy was soon extinguished when they came home with some very tedious birds. Not quite what I had in mind. To me, birds are not great pets. Okay, they can be quite pretty to look at but seriously, all they do is sit and chirp. So, so dull. You cannot take them for a walk. They do not fall in love with you, and they definitely do not play fetch. I was stuck with these boring birds for years. Then when I was married, I shared my dream with Saeed that I might one day have a gorgeous little pug. Their squishy faces are so utterly adorable! Though I knew he had had pet dogs himself, I never thought I would actually be lucky enough to have one of my own.

It was the night before my twenty-fourth birthday, and I was getting ready to celebrate. My life was going well. I was newly married, I just kickstarted my career, and I felt successful. Therefore, this birthday felt kind of special to me. Plus, I was looking forward to celebrating my first one with my husband. That day, I got back from work earlier than he did, and I was waiting to see what plans he had concocted to help me celebrate when I heard the key in the door. Well, I was utterly blown away when he walked in carrying the most incredible pug-shaped cake.

I was so happy that he had been so thoughtful. I felt my birthday could not get any better. I never would have expected what was about to happen. He turned around and walked back out again. I was a bit confused until he walked back in with an enormous box that I guessed must have many little presents inside it. But the moment I put my hand on it, I felt it move and I knew what he had done.

We had been married for about six months, but before then it had become our habit to visit pet stores. These visits had started a few days after our honeymoon. Usually, a new bride in our culture is expected to dress more extravagantly than usual. Therefore, when Saeed told me we were going out on the Friday just after we arrived from our honeymoon, I decided to wear one of my beautiful, lavish Moroccan dresses with an open abaya, matched it with a pair of high-heeled Louboutins, grabbed a cute clutch, and headed out the door without a clue where we were going. It was a fun outing, but I would have chosen flats if I had known where we were headed.

Saeed drove the car down into the Abu Dhabi port area and stopped by one of the small pet stores. I was thrilled to discover my husband had the same passion for pets as I did. I happily went from store to store playing with the cats and dogs. If you have ever worn super high heels, you will know how uncomfortable I was. The outfit really was not suitable for the smelly port area, but I was happy. On that day, we were not ready to take a pet home, but we visited those shops many, many times over the next six months as a kind of hobby. It was a fun time together.

Fast-forward to the night before my birthday and the enormous box. My hands were almost shaking with anticipation as I opened the lid, and I gave a little scream of delight to see a real live pug. When I pulled back the cardboard flaps, the cutest little smooshy face was looking up at me, and I fell in love immediately. It was the best gift anyone had ever given me, and I thought I would never be happier.

Names Matter, Whether It's a Baby or a Pet!

One of the first things to do when you get a pet is give it a name. That sounds like so much fun but, trust me, naming something is not easy! It is a big responsibility. That creature will be stuck with that name for the rest of its life so it has to be something good that you know you will not be embarrassed calling on the street. That is when it is a pet, so what about when it is a baby you are naming? That is a responsibility bigger than anything you can imagine. I always say that if there were two things children could blame their parents for when they grow up, they would be the name they are given and the quality of education they were provided. However, this section is about my pet, not my baby! But having undergone this exercise of naming something was good practice before getting pregnant!

My first thought was to call my pug "Mops" after Marie Antoinette's pug. Did you know she had a pug? It is true. Despite the way things ended for her, the woman had style. Saeed and I were lucky enough to enjoy a beautiful tour of her castle, Petit Trianon as well as visiting the impressive Château de Versailles on our "second" honeymoon, about a month after coming back from Maldives. Marie Antoinette's life was beautiful in many ways before the revolution, and I felt an affinity for her when I discovered she also loved my favorite type of dog. But I wanted to see what other options would be suitable for that squishy face.

After creating a long list to choose from, one name came out on top. Chai. This name was spot on. Chai's coat was a gorgeous fawn color, just like chai tea, and his nature was as sweet as the drink too. It seemed like the perfect name. I felt like I had achieved a significant milestone in dog ownership. But there were far bigger challenges ahead.

My gift from my awesome husband was possibly the most thoughtful, caring gift I had ever had in my life. I know Saeed wanted to give me something I would love, and I am honored that he would do that for me, but I was completely caught off-guard as I had never looked after a real pet before. Birds do not need much looking after. Clean their cage (so gross), a bit of bird seed each day, and a visit to the vet once a year, if they live that long, is about it. But a dog is an entirely different story.

I quickly found out I needed to learn what temperature a room should be for a dog, how to clean a pug's ears and wrinkles, how to set up its bed, which kind of bedding is best, and where the bed should be. I learned how often to take it outside to do its business and how often it needed to be fed. I looked up the kind of food that is best for a pug and everything a responsible owner could think of. But still. Reading about it is one thing. Doing it is quite another! Just like when you are having a baby, you need to learn all about bathing, soothing, feeding, and all that jazz. Learning to care for a pet, I would say, was not very different from taking care of a baby.

When your baby arrives, you will begin a journey of teaching your child about every single thing there is to know about life including how to eat, drink, and poop. It is so funny seeing a baby startled by its own hiccups, sneezes, or farts! A newborn infant is utterly dependent on you and helpless to do anything for itself. My experiences with my dog were definitely useful training for parenting, which is good because my birthday was about to get even more exciting.

Happy Birthday to Me!

Without a shadow of a doubt, hand on heart, I can say that my twenty-fourth birthday will always be the most special of my life. After a wonderful evening, I woke up early the next day to walk my new puppy, Chai, which was a wonderful way to start things off at 4am. I took Chai out in the cool of the pre-dawn light with the thought growing in my mind that maybe something even more special might be starting. And I was right. A quick trip to the bathroom and I realized I had a birthday gift from God: a positive pregnancy test. It was so much fun to hide the test in my bathrobe's pocket and surprise my husband! It was one of those truly magical moments Hollywood tries to recreate in its movies. We were starting a family of our own!

As we were there in the living room basking in our newfound joy, my little pug wanted to join in. Chai was dancing around our feet. But as his gorgeous little face looked up at us, he sneezed. He was sick! And so was I, with a stinking cold. I felt miserable. Of course, we were not going to take any risks after my discovery, so Saeed decided I should not go to work and took me to the clinic instead as a precaution. They checked me over thoroughly and suggested simple rest and good hydration would see me through. We headed home. But pets are a responsibility and Chai was sick, too. We took him to the vet to see what was wrong. The answer was everything.

Poor little Chai had an ear infection, skin infection, intestinal worms (gross, I know), and an airway abnormality. We learned that pet shops are probably not good places to buy animals. Who knew?! We discovered that the animals there are often the products of puppy farms, where the creatures are kept in dreadful conditions and infections are rampant. Chai was one of the unfortunate ones who, even at his young age, was suffering from poor care. Saeed immediately wanted to return him to the store, but that would not help him get better. Chai had joined our household and I wanted to take care of him until he was cured. Saeed appreciated my need to care and agreed. At the vet office, they started the treatment with a couple of shots, but it felt like we bought every medicine in the place to treat him! Our bag rattled with tablets. He may have had a bad start in life but then he found us, and I was hopeful he would make it through.

After I returned to work the following day, my husband called me. He had thought about the matter some more and had decided it was right after all to return the dog to the store. He did not want to put our unborn child at risk. I do wonder if things would have been different had we gotten Chai after having a baby because one thing is for sure, babies poop more than any dog. And dogs can be trained much more quickly than babies to do their business in the right place and at the right time! But the day after my birthday, Saeed didn't know all of this and his focus, quite rightly, was on the new life growing in my womb. I was heartbroken to lose Chai, my much longed-for pug, so soon after getting him, but I understood he was being taken away because something else was coming my way. This book is about that journey.

One thing I have learned on my journey into motherhood is that God gives, but he also takes away. What I learned from having Chai is that you might not always get what you want in life, but you can be sure that this is because God has something better waiting in store for you. Chai was taken away from me abruptly, but my first sweet child was growing in my womb. And I know which one I would rather have any day of the week.

Chapter 3
Before the Birth

The moment you discover you have a new life growing in your belly is one of the most magical moments you can experience, especially the first time. It's also rather terrifying. And, it's unfortunate that it typically happens in a bathroom in a rather undignified position... But hooray for modern medicine and peeing on a stick!

From the moment the second line turns blue on that pregnancy test, you are responsible for another life. The decisions you make about how you live can affect them, and your life will never be the same again. It's impossible to explain how profound parenthood is until you experience it. But if you're reading this book and your pregnancy test was positive, welcome to the club!

With such precious cargo on board, you need to be sure you're doing all the right things and that your pregnancy is going well. For this reason, it's so important that you find a good obstetrician. Some people will just find the nearest one or even Google "best obstetrician in Abu Dhabi" (just as I did). If you have time to visit a few, do so. Google is always the best place to start your search for anything, even something as important as a physician, though you have to be careful about what you find, and follow up with some real-world research of your own! You will know when you walk in if it's the right place. For me, what really matters is my own comfort. I want to feel well looked after, for the staff to pay attention to me, and let me in to see the doctor on time, and for the facility to be very clean and organized. In short, they need to come across as very professional.

I didn't want to have the most popular doctor or clinic. That is not the most important thing for me. If they are very popular but their clinic is a dump, I don't want to go there. They should care about their presentation, have the right staff to keep the place looking good, and most-importantly, they should not overbook patients in. If they don't care about these details, how can you trust that they care about you? Happily, I found one clinic that was perfectly clean, and it was right near my home in the city. Perfect! It looked good in the pictures and when I spoke to them to make the appointment, they seemed professional and their doctors seemed professional as well. So I chose one doctor, made an appointment, and I went to see her.

When I got to the clinic, I knew I had made the right decision. Everything was perfectly clean, there were flower arrangements, and I felt like it was a professional medical center. While I waited for my appointment, the staff checked on me to make sure I was okay, and they took me to see the doctor on time. If things hadn't gone so well, I would have walked out and found someone else. Don't be afraid to look around and find the right person. You have time at the start of your pregnancy to get this right and you don't want to regret your choice. It's the first major decision you will make in the care of your child, but it certainly won't be the last.

Here are four things to think about when choosing your obstetrician:

- Follow Up:

Will your obstetrician monitor you during the pregnancy and help you deliver your child, or will you need to find a different doctor for delivery? I liked to have the same person throughout, but for others that is less important. Ask this question at your first appointment or you may be disappointed later on.

- Birthing Choices:

Does your obstetrician support all the pain-relief options during delivery that you hope to have available to you? See my chapter on birth to learn why this is important!

- Comfort:

Are you comfortable at the clinic? Environment affects how we feel, and you should keep your stress down during pregnancy. What is your first impression of the clinic? Do they treat you well?

- Recommended:

Has it been recommended? If you have friends or family nearby who recently had children, ask them who they saw. Check to see if they were happy with the service they received. A good recommendation can save you a lot of time and is very reassuring. But make sure the person who is recommending has the same standards as yours!

Choosing the Right Clinic or Hospital

I know I said my comfort is very important to me. And I think it's really important that a doctor's clinic is clean! But the doctor has to be the right one, someone who checks all your boxes.

When I walked in, I got a reassuring, bright, and friendly first impression. The doctor was in her late thirties to early forties, and looked calm and confident. She smiled at me and introduced herself. I told her about my positive at-home test, and she took bloods to confirm the pregnancy. The obstetrician I had during my first pregnancy was really skilled at making me feel looked after and confident throughout the term. During my first meeting with her, she assured me that she would look after me well during my pregnancy. And this was the biggest thing for me. If she promised something or made an appointment, it happened when she said it would. With this doctor and the quality of the clinic, I knew I had found the right care for me and my child.

The place I chose was a private clinic, as opposed to government-owned healthcare provider. The main reason I chose a private clinic was to make sure I saw the exact same doctor every time instead of whichever doctor was on duty as done at public hospitals and clinics. And so, just as I hoped, I did all of my follow-ups with the same doctor throughout my pregnancy. Continuity of care is very important as the doctor will be well placed to notice if there are any developing issues over time and will know your medical history better than if you see different doctors each time. The only thing I would have changed is that this doctor did not attend deliveries. She was an obstetrician, yes. But her role was to only scan and monitor throughout the pregnancy to ensure the health and development of the fetus. If I could go back in time, I would have the same doctor that I chose to see throughout my pregnancy deliver my baby as that would have made me more comfortable.

Prodded, Poked, and Scanned

If you've never had anything worse than the flu or a broken bone, you might be surprised to find out how often you need to see your doctor throughout your pregnancy. From the time the second line on your home testing kit appears, you are beginning a new relationship, and I don't mean with your growing baby. I mean with your obstetrician who you will see every two weeks, on average! Here are the basics:

Before you get pregnant, you think of pregnancy in terms of "nine months." This isn't technically quite right, as months vary in length. So doctors talk about weeks of pregnancy, and a full-term pregnancy is forty weeks long. If you're not keeping track or actively trying to become pregnant, you're not likely to find out you're expecting until you are a few weeks along.

Here's what to expect from your first appointment:

They will ask you basic questions about your health and menstrual cycle. They will want to know about your family's medical history, in case there are any medical conditions they need to be aware of, and they will take some blood to confirm the pregnancy. They may even scan you. This won't reveal anything about the baby, as it is still just a small collection of cells at this point. But they need to check in case you are more pregnant than you know, and they will check the shape of your uterus and so on. It's no big deal but it will help them know how best to look after you and whether they need to see you more often than usual.

During the 12 weeks scan, a lot of measurements are taken. You may even find out at this point that you're expecting twins! Don't worry, though. For most parents, this scan is just a nice opportunity to get a first look at their child.

But don't bother asking if they can tell if it's a boy or girl yet, as those bits haven't developed enough to tell you! The 12 weeks scan is one of the most important ones done during your pregnancy as a lot of measurements are taken to detect chromosomal abnormalities in a fetus. So try not to miss this one! Just make sure to mark the calendar with the help of your doctor for scans that must be done at a certain point during your pregnancy to ensure that none of them is missed.

Some people choose to have a scan at sixteen weeks. It might be possible to discover the gender at this stage. We found out we were expecting a girl, though a friend was told the same at sixteen weeks only to be told at twenty weeks it was a boy, so don't go filling the nursery quite yet! You'll also have more blood tests around now. These check lots of things, such as anemia, glucose, and for abnormal chromosomes.

Another important scan during your pregnancy is called "the anatomy ultrasound" or "anomaly scan" and it is done at around 21 to 22 weeks of pregnancy. The objective of this ultrasound is to take a close look at your baby and to ensure that the baby's development is normal.

Your obstetrician is likely to take blood and urine samples around this time to check for diabetes, which can happen as a temporary condition during pregnancy.

Your doctor will be keen to check your blood, urine, and blood pressure as they keep an eye on signs of some of the main pregnancy conditions and some of the main disorders that can be detected from your blood, such as chromosome disorders. Most of the time the results are fine, but it's important to get the checks done when the doctor recommends them.

But don't worry, the hospital or the clinic will sort out all your appointments for you to make sure you don't miss any of the important scans.

Strap in for Your Hormone Roller Coaster

So what is it like being pregnant? Lots of books teach you about the baby, but it's just as important to learn about what's happening to you and your body. Some big changes are starting to happen. During the first couple of months of my pregnancy, I was quite emotional. I used to cry for no reason at all, then when I was done weeping, I would laugh at myself! It was so funny to me, but I totally needed to get those tears out of my system. It's true that a good cry can make you feel better—well, at least in pregnancy it can. When I first joined my workplace, I was only a few weeks pregnant. Not long after I joined, they had a farewell gathering for one of the employees and guess what? I started crying when I didn't even know the guy. He even gave me a look, which roughly translated as "Excuse me, have we met?" I'm sure my colleagues started calling me the crying girl, but what was I to do? Those tears needed to come out! It helped me decide to tell my boss and colleagues that I was pregnant very early on. I didn't want them thinking I was totally crazy.

Which brings me to my next piece of advice: pregnancy hormones can make you seem like an insane person, so you might want to announce to people that you're pregnant from Day 1!

That said, I understand that many people prefer to keep it a secret until the first trimester is over (12 weeks) in case of miscarriage. Despite the fact that I had a miscarriage with my third pregnancy at seven weeks, I am still a strong proponent of announcing a pregnancy early on. One of the main reasons I tend to announce is because I want to make those who care about me happy. Another reason is because I immediately start having attitude problems!

Fast-forward from my first pregnancy in 2014 to my third in 2019.

Miscarriage

After waking up soaked in blood, I drove myself at 3 in the morning to the hospital, thinking I am not alone and that the child growing inside of me was still there. I was still in denial as tests were being run. *It's all good*, I told myself. *Bleeding does occur during the first trimester, and it is absolutely normal*, I repeated in my head. But as the doctor came back two hours later with the result and said "I'm sorry!" I found myself reassuring the doctor that I was okay while she was explaining to me what had happened. "It's okay," "it's fine," "okay, thanks," "no problem," I repeated with a straight face while she was still talking, because on the inside, I just wanted her to stop. To go. To leave me alone.

I did not know how to process my grief. I felt vulnerable and alone until I spoke openly about it on social media the next day and found out that at least five of my friends had been through miscarriage as well. Why are we told to keep things like this to ourselves? "Do not tell anyone that you're pregnant. Beware of the evil eye." "Do not tell anyone that you had a miscarriage."

"Why?" I asked. But the reason was not disclosed! I am a believer in counting God's blessings every day, and speaking about them, and being pregnant is truly a blessing. That's why I choose to break the requisite three-month waiting period before announcing a pregnancy. I always announce on the day that I find out because happy news is meant to be shared with loved ones. I am also a believer in putting feelings into words, whatever they may be. Talking about what I went through made me feel closer to those who care. It made me feel better.

Are You Buying Blue or Pink?

Where did this cliché come from? I don't know. But I learned that pink was the traditional color for boys in Victorian England, so the whole thing has changed over the years. These days everyone buys everything blue for boys and pink for girls, as if there aren't any other gorgeous colors a baby could wear! As we had bought a beautiful blue baby Dior bottle, we really wanted to know the sex of our child. The funny thing is that I was under the impression that my baby was a boy ever since I found out that I was pregnant with my first. My husband was also eager to find out, so he bought a home gender test when I was a few weeks pregnant. He woke me up in the morning with a smile on his face, handing me that test to take first thing, before getting ready to go to the office. He was that eager! So I took the test and it showed that I was having a boy. So there I was, convinced from that moment onwards. What I didn't know was that obstetricians can't usually confirm the gender until around sixteen to eighteen weeks of pregnancy, or I wouldn't have taken this waste-of-money test!

For me, when the doctor told me that I was pregnant with a girl, I was shocked and started crying out of happiness. The doctor actually thought that I was crying because I did not want a girl and started saying things like "you can buy girls cuter outfits than boys." I was so shocked. Did she really think I would be upset about having a girl? It was horrific to think some people would react that way and be upset about having a girl. I did not really care what gender the baby was, as long as they were healthy. Having a baby is a blessing, and one should never be picky about what blessing we receive.

And that baby bottle? It went into one of my keepsake boxes. Looking at it always brings a smile to my face as I remember that time in the early days of our marriage.

People Love to Give Advice (Even When They Don't Know What They're Talking About!)

When you're pregnant, it is an exciting but scary time. You know your body is designed for this task, but some people find it hard to accept the idea of another life growing inside them. One way you can become more comfortable with your new pregnancy is to get good advice. But the problem is, you may well end up with too much of a good thing. Everyone, and I mean everyone, has an opinion for you when you're pregnant, and most of the time they're not afraid to tell you even if you don't ask. I came across what felt like a million different people with different opinions about what expectant women should or shouldn't be doing.

From my experience, I also noticed how much our society thinks it should tell us how to behave as well. Some people think that we are all China dolls who should do nothing more than lie down when we start having a bump, because any little thing we do can harm our growing babies and us. Hello? Have they tried talking to their own mothers and grandmothers? These women kept house as well as looked after their children and husbands before we had electricity or things like dishwashers and washing machines. They didn't let pregnancy stop them!

I did get a little frustrated by all the conflicting opinions, and so did some of my friends. What's funny is that many women who were hardworking in the past have been swayed by the general opinion of the society. The same women who used to milk cows and camels with their pregnancy bumps in a previous generation now tell us we should do nothing more than lie down! One of my friends was told by her older relatives to stay at home, not to move very much, and to eat a lot. But her younger friends told her the complete opposite: she should go out as much as possible, to see things and enjoy life before the baby comes and the crying starts.

Today's women know that our lives are different from the women who went before us, and we know that some people's advice comes from experience, but their experience is not ours. While you can try to get advice from books instead of well-wishing elders and peers in order to avoid engaging in endless arguments, you will find, as I did, that the advice in those books comes from places with different climates, different cultures, and different lifestyles, and must therefore be taken with a healthy helping of caution and common sense. And when in doubt, always speak openly to your doctor.

For example, I became a health and fitness enthusiast before my first pregnancy. I went to the gym daily for sessions with my trainer, and I saw no reason why this should stop simply because I was growing a baby in my womb. Some advice went against this, but I knew my body and my level of fitness was high. Happily, my trainer agreed with me. We decided that we would adjust my exercise routine if anything became too difficult because of my changing shape, but otherwise we carried on. Our plan was to listen to my body and not push it if there were any negative signals. And I'm glad we did. Toward the end of the pregnancy, I did slow down and there were some exercises my bump decided I couldn't do, but I didn't give up altogether.

So, What Should We Do and Who Should We Listen To?

If my friends and I listened to the advice we received when we were pregnant, we would have all been wrapped in cotton wool and protected in a motionless bubble throughout our pregnancies. If women had actually lived by that advice throughout history, I don't think the human race would be here now! Pregnant women have to be fairly tough, or how would the human race have survived so well in the desert or back in the days of prehistory?

To give you some idea of how things were when my mom was young, you might be shocked to know she got married when she was twelve. But in those days, this really wasn't unusual. The tradition used to be that the minute a girl got her period, she was ready to get married. I think this went on until the 1970s, when this country was formed. As Bedouin culture mixed with other cultures, we became more inclined towards cultural globalization and the government drafted laws regulating things like marriage. After that, it was illegal to get married before you turned eighteen.

In my mom's day (late 60s), it wasn't uncommon for women to have eight to ten children. My mom had eight; my mother-in-law had ten—that was the average back then. I cannot even imagine how exhausting it must have been to be a parent, especially at such a young age. But that was how things were done.

Women also did all the housework themselves. They didn't have help, not like now with housemaids. On top of that, because of the way traditional Emirati culture was half a century ago, women would regularly have lots of visitors to their home, whether or not they were pregnant. So there was always a lot of cooking and cleaning to be done along with taking care of all of the children at the same time.

Cooking, cleaning, and entertaining guests are not easy jobs. Women were expected to do these throughout all of their pregnancies, by themselves, as teenagers, without maids or nannies. In stark contrast, the modern practice of coddling pregnant women is not only quite ridiculous, it also certainly doesn't suit me.

As I listened to more and more "well-meaning" advice, I resolved not to listen to such nonsense and continue to keep fit and go out as I wanted, no matter what my elders and peers said.

The other big difference between my mom's youth and mine is that these days, of course, families want their daughters to complete their degree before they get married. That's what happened with me. I got married when I was twenty-three, right after graduation, and I became a mom at twenty-four. I've been observing a recent trend of first-time moms starting even later than I did. I recall recently four or five girls in my circle who did not get married until they were older than thirty-five. In the olden days, such women would have been talked about, called "aaanes" (spinster), and were cruelly teased.

Thankfully, this mindset is now considered old-fashioned, and the attitude toward women is finally changing. It's more about waiting for the right guy to come along and pursuing a career.

Of course, all of these changes and evolutions mean women are having fewer children. We see women getting married up to more than twenty years older than just a single generation ago, and the birth rate now is probably around four or five children per family if not less. I would predict that as the marriage age rises and attitudes toward women change even more, families could well start to have only one or two children each, like a lot of Western countries. Women also have more responsibilities now outside the home. Lots of women I know have children, a home, a career, and a side business while the tradition of entertaining friends and family in the home on a weekly basis remains strong. Who can do all of that with ten children around?

Staying in Shape

Our lives are very different from our mothers', but we need to ensure we stay fit now that we no longer have such physical work to do around the house. One week before finding out that I was pregnant with my first child, my trainer set me up with an interval training plan that would challenge anyone. But I nailed it!

When I found out I was expecting, my plan was to continue working out during the whole forty weeks of pregnancy. I gave my trainer a book about exercise called *How to Exercise When You're Expecting: For the 9 Months of Pregnancy and the 5 Months It Takes to Get Your Best Body Back* by Lindsay Brin. My trainer used to study the material every night and make me do the exercises the next day, right after I left the office. I was feeling healthy, light, and extremely comfortable with my pregnant body. The first four months of pregnancy went smoothly.

Before I got pregnant with my first daughter, working out was extremely easy to fit into my schedule. It felt really good. But life became too busy, and became even more so now that I have two daughters. For a while I worried about the weight, but I realized that the aspirational images we see in the media are all unrealistic. In time, I came to recognize that I am curvy. My body shape is curvy and, actually, I love my body. It has done amazing things like growing babies and giving birth. Because of social media and the unrealistic images we see, some people might categorize me as "fat." But I don't see myself as fat. I am proportional. I still carry a few extra pounds that I gained from the two pregnancies, but it's not something that troubles me anymore.

Like every other real woman who has a baby, I found out that it's really hard to lose the last few pounds. Birth control doesn't help. I certainly don't have ideas of getting extreme makeovers, like having a bypass surgery or liposuction for instance, although they're becoming a trend now and I know a lot of people who got them. If I'm going to have more children in the future, the weight is going to come back anyway. Plus all surgeries have risks. As long as all of the weight is going to come back, why should I do anything drastic like that now? I believe it is far healthier to just learn to love my body and exercise as much as I realistically can. I don't exercise or eat right in order to slim down to the size and shape of a model. I exercise because it makes me happy. I exercise because I like being healthy: for stamina and for endurance.

Bye Bye Toes

One thing most pregnancy books don't warn you about is the way your body is going to change, or the way you're really going to feel about those changes. Your belly may be lovely and flat when you start, but sharing and stretching that space with a new person is going to rearrange your shape quite a lot. Possibly forever. Of course, it's completely worth it, but we can all grieve for our flat bellies. What you shouldn't do is believe the images of celebrities with super-flat bellies weeks after they've had their baby. Remember Photoshop exists, and even if the Instagram posts are true, what you don't see is the hours those women spend in the gym while their body is still recovering from the birth, which is such a silly thing to do. Doctors say to wait at least six weeks for a reason. Also, those women have private chefs, personal trainers, on-call nannies, and night nurses. Celebrate the amazing thing your body is doing—growing a new person—and celebrate your new soft curves that your baby will love snuggling into after he or she arrives. A friend of mine calls her belly her "squishy mommy tummy," and her little girl adores resting her head on it when they cuddle. It's a much healthier attitude than starving yourself back to the shape you were in before. One day, you'll be in the right frame of mind to get yourself fit and healthy, and you can enjoy introducing your child to exercise in a positive way then.

Pregnancy Stages and What's Happening to You

The first trimester (Weeks 1 to 12) can be a tough time for many moms-to-be. You don't look pregnant, as your bump hasn't developed, but you may feel dreadful. Many women experience morning sickness. Some, like England's Duchess of Cambridge, become so ill with this that they cannot eat or drink anything and need to stay in hospital until it passes. It sounds awful, and I'm so sorry for you if it happens. Different women are affected by their pregnancies in different ways.

Other women may find they cannot eat or drink their usual favorites because they suddenly detest the smell or the taste. This can even go so far as to affect their reaction to random things like laundry detergent or their husband's aftershave. One woman I know had to go along the aisle in the supermarket sniffing each and every fabric softener until she found one she could tolerate! Other friends have had to give up coffee or tea, and stop eating spicy food and other things they used to enjoy regularly. A good friend of mine was lucky, as all her pregnancies went well. She didn't suffer from morning sickness or mood swings. She did, however, hate certain smells such as the smell of meat. Before she was pregnant with her son, she and her husband would often go to a particular Azerbaijan restaurant, but once she was affected by smells, just passing by it made her nauseous. Even today, she still remembers the smell of it and how ill it made her feel.

That same friend found she often felt exhausted when she was pregnant, which she hadn't expected. It doesn't help that here in the UAE, the climate is extremely warm. Some women can experience absolute fatigue and exhaustion. Apparently, this is because of the placenta in the first trimester. Think about it. Your body is literally growing an entire new organ in the pace of a few weeks! No wonder it can be a bit draining. The heat can make these feelings even worse, causing pregnant women to feel faint or dizzy, so air conditioning is essential. If this happens to you, make sure those around you understand what is happening, but take comfort from the fact that, for most women, these symptoms get better or even disappear at around twelve to fourteen weeks. When she was pregnant, my friend also remembers enjoying eating all the food she wanted without anyone frowning at her. There is a lot of pressure on women here to overeat during pregnancy. (Although with her second pregnancy, she suffered from gestational diabetes and had to carefully monitor her food intake.) In fact, we really don't need to "eat for two" when we're pregnant. Simply listening to our bodies and eating sensibly is all that's needed.

I did not experience any of the usual early pregnancy symptoms and was able to maintain a healthy, active lifestyle each time, thank goodness! During my first trimester, I felt absolutely ecstatic. I did not get any food aversions or morning sickness. Seeing what happened to people I know, I appreciate how lucky I was, but I do believe it's partly because I was living a healthy lifestyle. I believe that if one's body is used to doing a certain activity, stopping this activity suddenly would enervate it, and that is exactly why I did not want to stop my exercise routine. However, when people heard that I was still working out, they felt they had to tell me how wrong I was. I was bluntly told that I was going to kill my baby in the womb if I kept being so active. I still cannot believe how rude people were.

Comments like this about how I was living were not uncommon. It surprised me, as I hadn't experienced such rudeness before. It was like I suddenly became public property just because I was expecting a baby. People were telling me all sorts of dubious things, such as going on long rides is bad for the baby and riding in a Mercedes G Class (my husband's car back then) would lead to a miscarriage because of how bumpy it is on the road! Honestly, some of the things people came out with were utterly ludicrous. Things like exercising is bad for the baby, walking is bad for the baby, driving is bad for the baby. As if babies are connected only by a thread in the uterus and any movement will cut that thread and make me go into early labor. Of course, I ignored all of this nonsense throughout the forty weeks and decided to listen to my body and follow common sense, and so should you.

This is why my very first piece of pregnancy advice is to listen to your body, do your own research, talk with your doctors and nurses, and make up your own mind, instead of listening to insane advice from other people who have no medical training. This leads to my second piece of pregnancy advice: do whatever it is that makes you happy as long as it does not harm the development of your baby. I did, and I am glad I did. I did not rely on other people's notions and decided to rely on my own extensive research every time I doubted something related to my pregnancy. My first child was the best birthday present I have ever gotten. I had to take care of her, sure, but I also wanted to enjoy my pregnancy and not feel deprived of living my life normally.

In a nutshell, everyone will decide to tell you how to behave when you are pregnant. Listen to your doctors and your body and do your own research, whether by reading books or online articles. Now that you're about to be the mom, you need to start making your own decisions for the health of your child.

Surprising Changes

During pregnancy, my personality changed drastically and I even started talking differently. I was never the kind of person who told inappropriate jokes. I was never the person who swore out loud. I would do it in my head if someone bothered me, but never out loud! I was never the kind of person who gave blunt comments. That all changed once I got pregnant, and the first person who noticed was my husband. I would drop a swear word if someone on the road was driving in a reckless way, I would drop a swear word if someone at the mall hit me with his shoulder while passing by, and I would drop a swear word if I was talking about someone who had bothered me that day.

Some people believe that the pregnant woman's personality changes to reflect the personality of the baby, which I think is total rubbish! If a child grows up listening to swear words and inappropriate language, he or she will automatically become someone who speaks in an inappropriate way. However, if I teach my child about what is appropriate to say and what is not, their words will never be impolite. That is how my parents raised me. What I was going through, however, can be described in one word: hormones!

One more thing that changed during my pregnancy was my style. I had always opted for classic pieces when it came to handbags, shoes, and colors. During my university days when I used to blog about fashion, those who followed my blog could tell that I was "that girl" who dressed up in classic Chanels and Diors. During pregnancy, though, I started experimenting with new things and following trends that suited me. I started appreciating contemporary designers and modern, sometimes funky, pieces. I started thinking of fashion as art, where every piece I wore had to be artistic in its shape, colors, and patterns. It had to be different from what was out there and different from what everyone else was wearing. If I were ever a *fashion hermit*, it would be from my first pregnancy onward and not back when I had that blog! Looking back now at my younger self's style, I feel like I dressed like a grandmother. Lady Dior, Birkin, Chanel flap bag, classic pumps, and diamonds at nineteen? A note to my dear daughters: if you're reading this, do not make the same mistake I made! I regret not dressing my age, which was kind of caused by a Blair Waldorf influence, which, if you were a Gossip Girl fan, you would know what I mean.

Food, Glorious Food

Food has always been a big part of my life. It is one of the joys of my life, and thankfully, that was also true when I was pregnant. I would never understand people who say they just eat for fuel. It makes me wonder if their taste buds are switched off. There is so much to enjoy from our diets, and we don't have to eat unhealthily to have an abundance of delicious things each day. That doesn't mean I'm a health freak all the time when it comes to what I eat and drink. In fact, ever since I first enrolled at the American University of Sharjah, I became a heavy coffee drinker! I don't know what university will be like when my children have grown up and reached the age of enrolling in college, but my school is still currently one of the toughest universities in the country, if not in the Middle East, to the extent that people immediately assume that you are a nerd if you tell them that you studied there. AUS turned me into a coffee fiend. We had multiple assignments to be submitted in one day, in addition to two or three quizzes besides midterms being scheduled at the same time. So that called for at least two Venti-sized cups of Americano per day!

When I got pregnant, I knew everything I ate and drank would also be consumed by my baby. From what I learned through reading many, many books, drinking one cup of coffee is not harmful. There is still no consensus on how much caffeine is safe during pregnancy, though. Once I found out I was pregnant, I decided it would be safer to stop drinking coffee as much as I used to. I do believe our bodies and our babies let us know what they need. Maybe it was the baby who didn't like coffee, and that was why I was not longing for those Americanos anymore.

And that wasn't the only way my pregnancy changed my diet. I started craving other stuff—other unhealthy stuff. The first thing I craved was Magnum chocolate ice cream. It had to be the kind with nuts on the outside and vanilla on the inside. I remember that we were in Al Ain the first time I asked my husband to get me some. Husbands can be so helpful when you are pregnant! The second thing that I craved was Pepsi. Yes, Pepsi! I had cut down on soft drinks two years before I found out that I was pregnant, as I kept reading they really aren't good for us. But the baby brought Pepsi back into my life! And not any kind of Pepsi. It had to be Pepsi in a glass bottle! I remember that my husband brought me a plastic bottle of Pepsi once, and I started to cry. This is what our hormones do to us as our bumps are growing.

My father-in-law came to the rescue. He used to bring me a box of glass-bottled Pepsi every time he visited. Another thing that I craved was Kinder chocolate. Just remembering that I used to eat ten fingers of those every day is almost unbelievable now. Oh, and also feta cheese! There is a belief that if a pregnant woman craves sweet things she is probably pregnant with a girl, and if she craves salty foods then it is a boy. Or maybe it's the other way around. Whatever it is, I don't really believe in that notion! I wanted both tastes.

Thankfully, I did not have an aversion to anything during the pregnancy, but I have heard several tales from pregnant moms about the bizarre foods they have had to avoid. One friend of mine could not eat lettuce! It became disgusting to her. Another one stopped liking tea, when it had been her favorite drink her whole life.

To support myself in my goal to be as healthy as possible during my pregnancy, I bought a juicer paired with a book that would tell me how each ingredient in a smoothie would support the growth of the baby. I have always watched what I eat and worked hard to keep my sugar level from rising since I come from a family that diabetes loves so much. I continued to count calories even during pregnancy, and did not think of my pregnancy as a free pass to indulge in everything, except what the baby wanted! I was trying to do everything by the book just so that I wouldn't mess things up. And the outcome was a healthy baby who lived inside my tummy longer than she should have, but we will come to that later!

Do not feel bad if your diet is not super healthy during your pregnancy. Sometimes the baby wants what it wants! Ask your doctor for a list of foods that can be dangerous during pregnancy, such as liver and raw fish, and definitely avoid those. Otherwise, simply try as much as you can to keep a good ratio of healthy whole foods with lots of greens and protein in your diet and you're golden.

Pregnancy Adventures and How Hyper I Get

I am a strong believer in listening to your body about keeping fit and eating well. It's something I've followed my whole life, and my trainer agrees with me. During my pregnancy, I decided I would continue to listen to my body and continue my life as I had. I love traveling, although my husband is not really a big fan, but we made lots of plans to see other parts of the world before we discovered my first pregnancy. We then decided that we would not let pregnancy stop us from putting itineraries together. Although the trip we took during my pregnancy was rather spontaneous, even for us!

When I was sixteen weeks' pregnant with my first, a sudden plan came together. I was bored at work one morning. The "Isra and Miraj" holiday was coming up, which would give us a long weekend. So I decided to look at trips on the Internet to all the exotic and exciting places we wanted to visit. I found one to Nepal that looked incredible. The trip was full of adventures, doing things I had only dreamed of. So before I knew it, the flight was scheduled and we had booked our tickets to go the very next day! Early the next morning, we were up and out the door heading off for a three-day trip to Nepal—the roof of the world.

Flying when you are four months' pregnant is no problem, as long as you don't have any health issues. All my appointments with my doctor had gone well, so we had no worries about the journey. Our flight was easy and comfortable, so it felt like almost no time at all before we were being driven from the airport to our hotel in a van that only minutes before had dropped Selena Gomez at the airport, or so the driver told us! It was almost evening in Kathmandu when we arrived, so we checked in to the hotel, had dinner while being entertained by Nepalese traditional dancers, and got a good rest before the real adventures began.

There are a few differences between the UAE and Nepal that are immediately apparent. The first major one is the landscape. We are used to big urban cities with skyscrapers, surrounded by miles and miles of desert and the ocean. In Nepal, the only things that scrape the sky are the mountains, and there is no sea for miles in every direction. Nepal is home to Mount Everest, the tallest mountain in the world. The UAE boasts a skyscraper that is 828 meters tall, but that doesn't even come close! Another big difference is that Abu Dhabi and Dubai are only 27 meters above sea level, while Kathmandu is a staggering 1,400 meters. That kind of difference can affect anybody's health, as the air is so much thinner. But, luckily, the thinner air did not affect me or my husband. As we enjoyed our meal at the hotel, we looked out at a skyline of wispy-cloud-topped mountains with snowy peaks. We couldn't wait to explore.

Our first adventure was a flight around some of the Himalayan mountains. If you are in Nepal, you must find a way to see Everest. I wasn't about to start climbing it, of course. Instead we took a two-hour flight in a rather shaky plane. This definitely wasn't a luxury international flight with comfortable seats. The plane rattled and creaked and the seats were sturdy but hard. Any discomfort proved worth it, though, when we first saw the magnificent ice-topped Mount Everest and its fellow mountains. It is truly magical to see something you have always heard of or studied. We were truly awe-inspired looking at the impressive sight. The feeling was overwhelming and the snow-topped mountains were indescribably beautiful to look at. The time flew past and our first Nepal adventure was over before we knew it. But it wasn't the craziest thing I did. Not by a long shot.

We checked out of the hotel and took a four-hour drive to Chitwan, the jungle side of Nepal. People don't always believe me when I tell them that I went on a three-hour-long elephant ride around the jungle on a real-life Dumbo when I was sixteen weeks pregnant. But it's true. Riding an elephant isn't anything like riding a horse, but you are very safe and the guides look after you. Saeed, however, was panicking the entire time. He didn't stop complaining until a tree branch hit him on the face while our elephant, which was carrying the both of us besides an Australian couple, was passing a narrow pathway in the jungle. It was like a scene from a cartoon and a sign that Mother Nature wanted him to shut up! So there we were, riding through a jungle at the top of the world, with who knows what kind of animals lurking in the undergrowth, and I couldn't have been happier. But even that won't raise your eyebrows as much as what we did next.

On our last day in Nepal, I was starting to feel a little sad that our adventure would soon be over, but this was drowned out by my excitement for our last big adventure. We took a challenging, four-hour ride to Pokhara where the blood vessels in my nose decided to expand and my nose began to bleed. This was the first of my pregnancy nosebleeds. The private car we rented did not have any tissues. We had to stop down the road at a mini mart—and when I say mini mart I mean a person standing in the middle of the road with a cart of products! Saeed got out of the car and went to buy a tissue box in a panic… and came back with toilet paper! Paper is paper, after all, and it did work to stop the nosebleed so we could continue our journey.

If you ever get the chance to go to Pokhara, I highly recommend it. There is a stunning lake surrounded by mountains, and it is the perfect place to try a new sport that gives you a unique vantage point… Paragliding!

You read that correctly. And yes, I was sixteen weeks pregnant, and no, not everyone should try it when they're pregnant. There are risks, but we can't live our lives dictated by what might happen or we wouldn't be living at all. In fact, to be able to go, I lied and signed a form saying I wasn't pregnant.

From that moment on, things began to happen that felt like signs that this could be a bad idea. First, our tour guide told us that we could not take anything with us up in the air. We had to unload our pockets and put everything in my handbag, which he promised would be safe with his friend. A girl on a motorbike then drove up, stopped, and asked for our belongings to keep them safe. I watched her wear my Hermès Herbag across her body and bike away. I thought I was never going to see that bag again! However, I was about to have the experience of a lifetime that no material thing could match.

At the time, I felt with certainty that my baby would be safe and sound inside me as I flew over the landscape with my instructor. Saeed was nervous but he trusted me. And wow. Paragliding over the landscape with the air rushing past your face almost as if you are a bird in flight is an incredible experience that I would love to do again. It was truly one of the most amazing things I've ever done, and I recommend it—but definitely after you've had your baby!

Saeed, on the other hand, started to panic when we were up in the sky, worrying that he shouldn't have let me do it because suddenly, he saw me flipping over! My instructor thought it would be fun to flip me over repeatedly before we landed. I must admit I feared experiencing a miscarriage in Nepal, so far from home and from the care I was familiar with. Even though that thought crossed my mind while I was high up in the air, I still managed to enjoy every second of it.

P.S. Do not go paragliding while pregnant and hold me responsible for it!

Getting Bad News About Your Baby

Not long after we returned from Nepal, I had reason to realize how lucky we are to have full health insurance, which gives us the luxury to choose between private and public hospitals where all the essential treatment is covered. Some moms-to-be in other countries don't have this luxury and when things go wrong, it's not only emotional, it can lead to bankruptcy (Thank you, UAE!).

I had no discomfort whatsoever in my first, second pregnancies, or fourth pregnancies (my third resulted in a miscarriage). Everything was going well. I didn't suffer from morning sickness, high blood pressure, diabetes, or any of the other conditions that can happen during the three trimesters. But one morning while I was at the office while pregnant with Shereena, my first, I had a call from my doctor's clinic. I'd been in for bloods a few days before, and the doctor wanted to see me. I didn't think anything of it until I was shown in to the examining room and I saw her face. She looked very serious.

The way she talked to me terrified me. Thank goodness Saeed had come with me, though he was scared himself. She told us that my blood seemed to have more chromosomes than normal, which meant there was a chance my baby could suffer from Down Syndrome. And that's when the weeping started. I was literally pinching myself, hoping that this was one of the pregnancy-caused nightmares that I had been having. She advised me to go see another doctor, someone more specialized in this field and who could give me a definitive answer. And we went to her office immediately. She was one of those doctors who gives you a sense of tranquility and reassurance from the moment she says "hello." I knew straightaway when I saw her that she was excellent, and the way she was explaining everything consoled me a little bit. She gave me three options:

- Option 1: To have another blood test done, which would be risk-free and would tell us with 99 percent accuracy whether or not our baby had Down Syndrome.
- Option 2: To have amniotic fluid sucked out of the amniotic sac with a needle, which could be tested and would tell us with 100 percent accuracy whether or not the baby had Down syndrome. This procedure, "amniocentesis," carries a risk of miscarriage which can vary depending on a variety of factors like maternal age and your medical history.
- Option 3: To let it go and not think about it and accept whatever God gave us.

The blood test, although the safest way to go, would have made me worry throughout the remaining four months of pregnancy. And as they say, worry kills! Although it is 99 percent accurate, I knew for sure that the 1 percent would drive me mad until I gave birth and saw for myself. Letting it go and not thinking about it meant that I could be choosing a hard life of abnormality for my child. Yet it was the one I wanted to choose. I believe in destiny. While I was contemplating the options, Saeed tried very hard to convince me to go for option 2. So I succumbed and I had the amniotic fluid tested.

They pushed a needle through the wall of my abdomen into my womb and pierced the amniotic sac around the baby. Saeed was holding my hand and I was squeezing it hard. I cried throughout the procedure. It was by far the most difficult thing I ever went through. When the needle started sucking out the amniotic fluid, it felt as if a balloon had been popped in my stomach. Right then, I thought my child was gone despite all the doctor's reassurances.

To lighten the mood after that traumatic experience, Saeed took me to Zuma, one of my favorite restaurants, for lunch. But that did not help me forget what we were in the middle of. I was gloomy and I barely ate anything.

We were told that the result was supposed to come out within five days, and if I did not suffer from any bleeding within three days, then the chance of miscarriage would subside. For those five days, I was in extreme desolation. I chose not to see anybody or talk to anyone. I took time off work. I was just lying down on my left side, which allows for maximum blood flow, crying into my pillow, reading about amniocentesis on different websites, and hoping for the best. I was trying as much as I could to focus on the positive feedback of women who had undergone the procedure, rather than any of the negative comments. It truly helps when you read the stories of people who have gone through what you have been through, rather than people who have no idea what this is about. Which is why Saeed and I decided not to tell anyone. We kept our worry and pain to ourselves until we heard the answer.

After five days, I got a call from my doctor very early in the morning, which made me stand up on the bed. That's how eager I was to know the truth! She knew how miserable I had been with worry, because I had called the clinic many times since the amniocentesis asking if the results were in.

She said that my baby was fine and that I had nothing to worry about. I cannot explain the sense of relief and happiness that I felt.

If you were to undergo a similar situation, and I hope to God you never do, always think positively and hope for the best. Never give in to fear.

Praying to God and hoping for the best can help a lot in comforting you during a period of fretfulness. Talking to people about your concerns can also help, especially people who have been through the same thing, but make sure you are talking to the right people and not ones who would make you worry more. Online support groups can be a great option. But if you feel that letting it out could weigh you down even more, don't! People sometimes worry with you and sensing their apprehension can make you feel worse. Turn to God and pray and everything will hopefully be okay.

Broken Leg While Pregnant

I flew back from Nepal so proud of myself for not letting my pregnancy prevent me from reaching my goals and trying new things. I felt on top of the world, but I was about to get a wakeup call and a big lesson on the realities of pregnancy.

I was heading home at the end of the day, exiting the building of my workplace, when a terrible thing happened. Something that I probably could have avoided if I had been walking slower like a pregnant lady normally would! It was a very hot summer day in the middle of August, and our building was extremely cold. Hot weather outside, cold air inside... it doesn't take a scientist to see that extremes like that can lead to condensation. The building did not have a proper ventilation system, which led to dampness on the floor by the automatic glass door. I remember saying goodbye to one of my colleagues, and the moment I turned my head—crash—I found myself on the floor. I had slid on the wet patch and instantly felt the most excruciating pain in my leg. My growing baby bump did not exactly help with stability.

A kind lady helped me get up and tried to walk me to the nearby sitting area. But we couldn't go anywhere. The pain was unbearable, and I could barely move my left leg. She sat me down and started performing first aid. But the more she tried to tilt my foot, the more I felt like kicking her from the excruciating pain.

I called Saeed and tried to sound normal so that I wouldn't scare him, but it didn't work. I told him that I couldn't drive and I needed him to pick me up. I can't imagine what his driving was like because he got to my office in half the time it should have taken him. My superman came to the rescue! The building's security guards brought a wheelchair and pushed me to the car and Saeed drove me straight to the hospital. Of course, he and I were both worried about the baby, not even thinking of what had happened to me as I was around thirty weeks pregnant.

When we got to the emergency room, the doctor explained it was highly unlikely my slip had hurt the baby, but he took the baby's vital signs just to be sure. Then he delivered the bad news. He could not order any X-rays because there was too much risk to the fetus. Without an X-ray, they couldn't confirm if I had a broken bone. It was a conundrum. In the end, the doctor on duty decided to assume that there wasn't a fracture, but he put a cast on anyway—just in case! Then he gave me an appointment to see an orthopedist in a week.

What choice did I have but to go home and stay in bed for seven long days until my appointment came around? It was depressing. I am the type of person who is very active, and staying at home with my leg up on a pillow or a table for a week was a nightmare for me. On the plus side, it gave me the perfect opportunity to watch loads of "Friends" episodes, especially the ones where Rachel is pregnant.

After seven arduous days, I went to the orthopedic appointment. As a positive person, I took the view that I was completely fine, the cast would be off that day, and I would be back at my desk before I knew it. The orthopedist knew more about X-rays than the emergency room doctor and decided I could have one as long as I wore a large lead apron covering my bump. It would protect the baby from the harmful X-rays, which after all, only needed to see my leg bones. And there it was: a fracture at the end of my shinbone around the back of my foot. That cast was going nowhere.

Anybody else would be pleased to learn they would need to stay at home and rest. The doctor wrote out notes for me and a letter for my employer. I cried when I saw he gave me forty-two days off. I loved my job. I loved feeling that sense of achievement and the routine that went with days at the office. I would finish work feeling good and then head to the gym for a healthy workout. Or I might have some errands to run and head across town. I might have arranged to see friends or go to a restaurant with my husband. Being stuck at home for a month and a half felt like a prison sentence. Even now, after three rounds of maternity leave and with my gorgeous children to play with, I hate being stuck indoors.

Doctor's orders were to have my leg raised on a pillow or table, and I was to avoid walking as much as possible. That didn't leave much room to do anything except watch TV, read, and go online. It was, however, quite good practice for being at home with a newborn. When you have a tiny person who needs to eat or sleep on an hourly basis, you can't get much done. If you're breastfeeding, you might feel like they're attached to you all day and night. So you will find yourself in a similar position to me with my leg. The best thing to do is to be prepared. Make lists of things you need to buy so you can search for some online bargains, and make a mental list of lots of shows to watch at your convenience.

My problem was that I hadn't planned to be stuck home at that point. I still hadn't really bought anything for the baby, apart from the gorgeous blue Dior bottle many months before, which I wouldn't be able to use because I was having a girl! So I did what I do best: I shopped online. Finding the best products can mean scouring the world, even with the exorbitant shipping fees. But I didn't care. If I had to be stuck at home, with no one for company and little to do, I was going to make the best of it. Hearing the doorbell chime delivering my wonderful packages gave me great joy and broke up the monotony of the day.

Another great solution when you're stuck at home and starting to feel blue is to take advantage of a home beauty service. When I was pregnant and my foot was in the cast, I treated myself to a manicure and pedicure, right in my own living room. It was a bit strange to make a pedicure appointment for one foot, but it worked for me! I thought it was cheeky of them to charge me full price, though. Of course, there are many other home beauty treatments you could try to cheer yourself up on a tough day. These are great when you're pregnant and also after the baby arrives. Many of my friends choose home service for facials, massages, or even eyelash tinting. The only difference between pre- and post-baby services is that after your little one is born, you'll need to pick a service that won't last more than forty-five minutes once your baby is home with you, as that's pretty much the limit of me-time you'll get for quite some time. You should also ask your beauty therapist to allow some extra time for your appointment in case you need to go and settle your baby. When you're childless yet pregnant, however, you may enjoy a treat like this in peace.

My husband did his best to lighten my mood as much as he could. He offered to take me out in a wheelchair so I could go to the malls. But we only went twice. I had to consider how exhausting it must be to push a pregnant lady around and I couldn't enjoy myself too much, knowing how hard it must be for him. It wasn't worth the effort and I enjoyed myself just as much cruising around in the car when he finished work. We were very sad to realize that the accident meant we weren't going to be able to fulfill our plans of celebrating each anniversary with a trip abroad. We had chosen to go to the Maldives again for our first anniversary and it was going to be very difficult with the pregnancy, but the cast made sure it couldn't happen. Saeed and I promised each other we would make it up with a bigger trip for our second anniversary, which we did by going to a beautiful resort in Maldives with a 10 months old baby.

With typical bad timing, but of course through nobody's fault, Saeed then had to accompany his father to Thailand for a medical checkup while I was still stuck at home with the cast. There was no way I was going to manage on my own for several weeks. Off I went to my parents' house for a little TLC from mom. It was lovely, actually, as she really took care of me. Sometimes it's nice to be the child, even when we are adults. Being back at the family home meant I also saw some of my brothers and sisters, and it turned out to be very sociable and a little like a real holiday.

Happily, my bone healed so well the cast came off in just a month, so I had twelve days' sick leave left before I had to return to work. The day after having the cast removed, I woke up finding Saeed in front of the mirror, getting ready for work. He asked me what my plan was for the day now that I could drive and walk. I kept thinking for a while until he said, "Why don't you drive to Dubai and meet up with your friends while I'm at work?" So like a caged animal whose door has just been opened, I took full advantage of my newfound freedom and fled. I drove straight to Dubai to meet up with one of my sisters for breakfast, then went to my family's house to chill for a while, then went to see my best friend, Noura. Noura and I could only hang out for a few hours, but we made every minute count; shopping, chatting, and having a great time. She admired my bump and couldn't believe what I told her about Nepal. I had to show her the pictures as proof. It was such a relief not having to hobble around with a big lump around my leg. Dubai was the perfect antidote to my recent confinement, and I didn't arrive home until really late at night, after Saeed had gone to sleep. I definitely made up for the long boring weeks in the cast, and I was ready to return to work.

I ended up going back to work about two months after my injury, which meant I was a little bit more than eight months' pregnant. To my amusement, after that incident, I was called "the girl who slipped downstairs" by my coworkers. Walking became a struggle with a healing ankle and swollen feet due to water retention during the last couple of months of pregnancy. However, I was still active. Especially after having to stay home for so long, the mood I was in, I could even have taken off on a hike across some beautiful scenery if only I had been allowed to fly and go somewhere far, far away! Being heavily pregnant put a stop to all that.

Strike a Pose: The Photoshoot

My last month of pregnancy with my first was a whirlwind. As well as working, I was finishing up all the books I had purchased and trying to memorize as much as I could about how to care for a baby, as if I was about to enter a final exam any second. I was also washing the baby clothes, ironing them, and arranging them in her little wardrobe. But my favorite task of all, which I advise every mother to do, was having a maternity photoshoot with a newborn and maternity photographer. Before we had the baby, she took amazing pictures of my husband and me in different outfits and different poses. A week after our child was born, we took her along for a photoshoot with the same photographer, and then she combined our pictures with the baby's in a beautifully made album. This is something I am planning to do for all of my pregnancies and all of my children. However, my third child, Alia, who was born during the COVID-19 pandemic was deprived from having a professional photoshoot. Instead, she is going to have a printed album of pictures taken using her mommy's mediocre photography skills, with iPhone quality!
Another keepsake that I put together during my ninth month of pregnancy with Shereena (notice how the first child always has more perks than the rest) was a sonogram photo album that shows how my baby was growing. This is something I have not done for my other children.

Let's Talk Books

One thing I wish all women do when they're pregnant is make sure they're well informed—not by listening to old wives tales but by getting the real knowledge from books. The best thing you can do for your unborn child is make sure you are well-educated about what is going to happen and what could go wrong. Being prepared is a huge step forward towards great parenting.

My knowledge about taking care of babies before I had my own was minimal if not zilch. My experience with my friends' and family's babies was limited. The minute they screamed or pooped, they were handed back. I had definitely been a hands-off kind of auntie. But, since information is power, the minute I found out that I was pregnant with my first child, I bought lots of books. During the pregnancy and over the first few months after having my first born, I read EVERYTHING!

To be fair, most of the books I read repeated the same information. But that was not a bad thing. Considering how clueless I was, it meant the most important things were reinforced and, as far as I was concerned, having all that information was going to help me make sure I kept my baby alive! But that's not the only reason I read so much: I will confess to being a teeny bit competitive. Every woman wants to be a good mom, but I was obsessed with being the best mom who had ever lived!

The books I devoured taught me everything I needed to know about what to expect during pregnancy, what I could do during labor, and how I would feel afterwards. I learned about how the baby was growing inside me, what it would want to eat and drink and when, how to dress her, help her sleep, and play with her. I learned about child development and what to look out for in case of problems. I found out more than anyone could ever want to know about giving birth, unless they're going to be a doctor or midwife!

Check Out Some Websites

Books weren't the only source of information I used. My husband and I registered with babycenter.com, a website that sends out a weekly email with information about the development of the baby in the womb. I would forward it to my husband, and we would sit together after work every Monday (the day we received the email) and talk about the child and how fascinating her development was. It was so special being able to share the journey with him like that. Men can often feel a little left out of the process during pregnancy. It's all happening inside your body, and they never get to experience that connection you get with your unborn child. Looking at those emails together was a great way to involve Saeed more.

Don't Forget the Videos

I'm kind of a visual learner. When I'm trying to learn something practical, it helps me if I can see a demonstration rather than just hear or read about it. A book with great illustrations makes a big difference in how much I remember and whether I remember it correctly over time. But watching someone giving a demonstration on film is definitely the best way to help me know what I'm supposed to do.

After reading a ton of books throughout the first pregnancy when I was stuck at home after breaking my ankle, I had a set of DVDs that were always, ALWAYS playing in my living room called "Laugh and Learn." I picked these out because I love things that are funny and their titles made me think they would be a fun way to find out about the practicalities of babies and birth. However, there is nothing to laugh about when it comes to the topic of childbirth. Thankfully, I didn't know that when I was thirty-six weeks pregnant! If you have time to fit it in, I recommend you get your own copy of the "Laugh and Learn" series. There is "Laugh and Learn about Childbirth," "Laugh and Learn about Breastfeeding," and "Laugh and Learn about Newborn Baby Care." I know that DVDs are pretty outdated, but I still purchase them! I kid you not, these DVDs cover everything from how labor works, to breathing techniques, pain relief, things the doctors can do to help, and what happens after the baby comes out. Sorry to say that isn't the end of the job. The new mommy still has a bit more to do before she can rest. My mantra is that a first-time mom-to-be can never have too many guides. So read and watch as much as you can! These DVDs were honestly very helpful. They basically refreshed my memory about the subjects I had read about before, and they illustrated many useful techniques and methods, which have been cemented in my head ever since!

Time for Yourself or for the Baby?

This is a debate pregnant women have had since they went out to work: When is the right time to start your maternity leave? For us in the UAE, maternity leave starts after the baby is born. However, a lot of us end up with a sick note from our doctor a few weeks before delivery or decide to take a few days of annual leave before the baby comes. My due date was the twenty-fourth of November. I worked up until the sixth of that month just to make sure everything was ready for my baby to come to this world. I would have worked up to my due date if I could have—even though my worst fear was having my water break at the office. That would have been very embarrassing. I would much rather be called "the girl who slipped downstairs" than "the girl whose water broke all over the office carpet!"

I kept working for a few reasons. As you know, I love my job and I wanted to show that I was still capable of doing it. No pregnancy and no broken leg were going to stop me. But also, I am a real get-up-and-go girl. I feel like I am wasting my time if I just lie down on the sofa doing nothing!

Maternity leave in the UAE is all right, I'd say! It's not the luxury of some northern European countries, who give women a year or more at home with their infants. When I had Shereena, the law was sixty days of maternity leave. When we put that together with annual leave, it gave me plenty of time to bond with my child, learn how to be a parent, start getting a routine in place, and find my feet. By the time I had my second daughter in 2017, the maternity leave in the UAE was extended and I could have three months off. That felt like more than enough. With my third child though, I had moved to a different company which had different maternity leave options that could extend up to six months: first two months with full pay, second two months with half pay, and the third two months without pay.

Being pregnant for the first time is new and strange. You are learning what your body is capable of, and you are experiencing things for the first time. Sometimes it can feel like an illness rather than pregnancy. With swollen ankles, a big belly, and poor sleep, you might think you need to use that maternity leave or the annual leave days you have as time to rest before the baby comes. And I totally get it. The problem is that if you use some of that time before the baby comes, you are likely to regret it afterwards.

I know that being heavily pregnant isn't easy, and you might feel you need to stop, but if you are able to keep working, try to do it. Of course, if there are medical reasons why you need to rest, just go home. Your doctor is the best person to help you decide what's right for you and your baby. But if the doctor says it is okay, save the maternity leave or your annual leave days to top up your maternity leave and spend more time with your new baby. You are going to fall in love in a way that has never happened to you before, and you will want to spend every minute you can with this wonderful new person.

Plus, I'm sorry to say that the lack of sleep in pregnancy is nothing like the lack of sleep with a newborn. You wouldn't want to hear this, but it really is harder after the baby arrives. You will need maternity leave to be able to rest during the daytime when your child is sleeping. If you have to go back to work too soon, you will be trying to cope with sleepless nights and doing a good job for your boss. Some people are lucky and have babies that sleep well, but who knows what your baby will be like? Most babies take around six months to become good sleepers. Speaking of which, did you know babies have to be taught to sleep at nighttime? They don't know what day and night are, so you and your routine have to teach them. If you're trying to do that and then head out to work a few hours later, you may find it too much to handle.

Everything I just said is totally different with later children. With my second daughter, the maternity leave felt very long and I got really bored! It had grown from sixty days to ninety. I know some people might be shocked, but I wanted to go back to my usual routine, back to working and talking to adults. With the first one, I felt like there were not enough hours during the day to know my baby and what she wanted. But with the second child, it felt like I had already done it all and I was ready to go back to my regularly scheduled life. We are so lucky to have that option these days. For our mothers and especially our grandmothers, once they had children, life at home with the baby was almost all there was.

Chapter 4
The Birth

The big day has arrived. Your water broke or your contractions have begun or your C-section is scheduled. Whichever way it begins, it's your baby's birthday and the day your life changes forever. Welcome to motherhood.

As you step into your third trimester, it is a good idea to put together a birth plan. There are many books full of advice about pain relief, positions, who to have with you, what to eat and drink, how to cope with contractions, and every other detail. But when it actually happens, you may well want to throw your plan away! However, that does not mean giving up on planning. If you have a birth plan with ideas about what kind of pain relief you want, what position you want, and whether you want things like a birthing pool, then your birth partner can help you get the things you have planned for on the day. You will be too busy having contractions to remember the plan yourself.

Birth is a very individual experience. Personally, I felt mentally and physically ready to embark on this new journey. I was just back from a morning shopping spree with my mother-in-law at the fish, fruits, and vegetables market. I came home, showered, and sat in front of the TV with some fresh pineapples that I purchased that morning. I was told that pineapples induce labor and thought of giving them a shot! At that time, I was forty-one weeks' pregnant and was supposed to see the doctor the next day to be induced. I felt somewhat wet and remembered my sister-in-law telling me about her friend who lost bladder control during pregnancy. I was afraid that's what was happening to me. I got up, took another shower, changed into a new set of clothes, and sat on my sofa once more with those pineapples. A few minutes later, I felt wet again! And I got up, showered, and changed into a new set of clothes one more time. I kept thinking my bladder control was no longer existent until I finally realized it wasn't my bladder—it was my water! My water did not "break," it just leaked. I had always expected that when my water broke, it would be like the movies—you know, like a giant water balloon had popped all over the floor. But not me. Not this time. Just like that, I was off to the hospital.

My husband and sister-in-law came with me to the hospital. If you are Western, going to the hospital with my sister-in-law may seem strange to you, but in the UAE we live with our husband's family after marriage and we can grow very close to our sisters-in-law. They become like our own sisters. On my way to the hospital, I texted my sister, Aysha, who drove to Abu Dhabi from Sharjah with my mother. Meanwhile, another support system was on the way from Dubai – my sister Wedad.

I remember arriving at the hospital feeling scared. I did not know what I was about to get myself into. While I was waiting for a nurse to take me to the ward, my husband was feeling hungry and asked me if I wanted anything from the vending machine. Seriously? There is a picture of us standing in front of the vending machine with him putting a strawberry milk carton and a chocolate bar close to my face. The look on my face in that picture is priceless—I was really furious!

One of my friends had a better birth experience than she predicted because she had thought about it beforehand and decided to follow her own choices on the day. She used yoga and swimming in the two months before going into labor to prepare her body for the birth, and it went well. As part of her preparations, she visited three hospitals but ended up giving birth in the same hospital she had been born in. Another friend had planned to deliver her child at a private hospital with a doctor she was seeing during the pregnancy. Her mother ended up taking her to a government hospital, and her husband wasn't even in the same city at the time. We can plan and plan how we want things to go, but on the day we have to accept that sometimes the environment decides things will be trickier for you. You might even end up with an unplanned c-section.

My plan was to give birth at the oldest maternity hospital in Abu Dhabi and the largest in the country. The reason behind my choice was that so many people told me that I should be in a well-established maternity hospital for my first pregnancy in case any complication arose during delivery. That same hospital is one of the very few with a neonatal intensive care unit, God forbid I would need it. I have heard stories about women who gave birth in private hospitals and right after delivery, they were transferred to a government hospital in an ambulance because the newborn needed to be in a NICU. The only thing that I did not like about this hospital, though, was that you could not choose your own doctor to follow up with during pregnancy and have the same doctor attend your delivery. Well, you can but you have to pull some strings and prove that you are a VIP for them to arrange that, something I hate and would never do! For "regular patients" like myself, whichever doctor is available will see you at your appointment, and whichever doctor is on duty will attend your delivery. Of course, if you have connections, you can definitely put whichever doctor you like on standby.

Your Hospital Bag

What should you take to the hospital when you go into labor? Besides the essentials, I packed my makeup because I am expected to look good when people visit, my hairdryer, my skin care products, my favorite perfume, my phone charger, and some fancy-shmancy maternity gowns. How you look when people come for the hospital reception is really important. People talk about it and there is definitely pressure from society to get this event exactly right. But more about that later.

For the baby, I packed some classic baby gowns that I wanted to put on my daughters when they were born. Personally, I don't like dressing them in overalls or onesies right after birth due to how difficult it is to change a newborn's diaper when in those. It is also important for the bellybutton not be chafed or restricted, which an overall or a onesie will definitely do. I picked up this habit from my mom, who used to dress us in these cotton gowns as well, with blue embroidery for boys and pink for girls. The baby also needs swaddles, hats, gloves, and socks. Do not worry about the diapers, as the hospital will give you enough to use during your stay.

Going Through Labor

While some countries are moving away from hospital-style managed births and toward natural births at home or in midwife-led centers, here in the UAE our trend is in the opposite direction. No one does home birth anymore, not since hospitals were established. Before hospitals became commonplace, the mortality rate for mothers and babies was rather high from what I hear, so understandably new moms want to have all that medical knowledge and help right there, just in case.

For most women, the news they're about to give birth arrives when they have regular contractions or their water breaks. In the weeks running up to the birth, you might feel some small contractions. These are called Braxton Hicks—but don't go running to the labor ward if you get them. Wait and see if they are regular or if they stop and go away. When you start having proper contractions—and trust me, you will know when they are proper ones—you will need to head to the hospital you have chosen. Remember to take your hospital bag, and don't race there in the car. A bumpy ride is no fun for a woman in labor. You will usually have plenty of time. Just keep in mind that first babies tend to take longer to get here than second or third ones.

Every birth story is a wonder and a horror at the same time. Yours will be unique to you, but we can all learn some good tips from other people's experiences. One of my friends was told to eat dates and keep walking when her contractions started before getting to the hospital. Of course, as the contractions sped up, this became impossible. But staying upright for as long as possible is supposed to help the baby move down the birth canal. Some people use a Swiss Ball to stay upright and feel more comfortable. It is like sitting on a squishy chair, which can help a bit. Sadly, swiss balls are not commonly provided at hospitals. Other people choose music or lighting that will be soothing. But how do you deal with the pain?

One of the girls I went to university with was a typical first-time mom. She was really worried and scared. Before the baby came, she kept asking everyone all the questions she could think of in addition to reading books and online articles and watching birth videos. All her close friends told her how painful it is, and everyone said that she should have an epidural. She agreed, saying, "I think that is the best choice for the first labor." But after having her firstborn, her legs were numb for a while and her whole body was aching. She had back pain for six months and she couldn't sit properly, which she believes was a side effect for the epidural. Medically, the only aspect of this that is likely due to the epidural is the leg numbness, which is just the anesthetic effect. It takes some hours for it to reduce and fade away. Potentially the back pain could also be from the epidural, but it is more likely that the months of being pregnant and then the birth itself actually caused this pain. That same friend decided she did not want an epidural with her second baby. Though, when it was time and she was experiencing powerful contractions, she found herself screaming for it. But, she reflects, "It wasn't bad at all. The pain was bearable and the birth went faster than my previous one. After having my second baby, I wasn't as tired as before. I could hold my baby and take care of him. The pain was just momentary. I also had a natural birth for my third child, and honestly I prefer it. I listened to my own instincts and took care of my children in my own way."

When your birth canal reaches ten centimeters' dilation, you will have to push. This is one reason why some doctors and midwives prefer not to give epidurals to first-time moms: you do not know what to push when you cannot feel it and you have never used those muscles before. Another friend ended up having a forceps delivery after her epidural, and her baby had big red marks on her head for a few days. This was because she didn't push well enough since she couldn't feel anything due to the epidural.

If you're having a natural delivery and you're fully dilated, your midwife might start screaming sometime around now. You are so exhausted that she becomes like the world's strictest gym instructor or sports coach. Do not be shocked if you get yelled at to push! It almost feels as if you are being humiliated in front of your family and the nurses! Most of the yelling happens if the baby is stuck in the birth canal, which can be very dangerous. In the past, many children and some mothers died during this stage, but don't worry! Today's midwives are trained to help you through it. Just attend to their instructions and do what they say, even if you feel too tired or like you don't have any energy left. Babies don't come out in a prescribed position each time. Sometimes they stick out their elbows or come out feet first. Midwives know the dangers and they know what they have to do to make the first-time mom work hard enough! So do not be surprised if your midwife jumps up on the bed with you and shouts in your face. It really is her job to be tough with you!

Another somewhat humiliating thing that happens when you give birth is that you give up your privacy simply because everyone wants to be there for you in case you need anything. While I was still in labor, everyone was in the room: my two sisters, my mom, my mother-in-law, two of my sisters-in-law, and my husband (before he decided it was a good idea to take a nap on the exit staircase). All these people were in the room along with the medical staff popping in and out. However, once the delivery started, I made sure that everyone was on the other side of the curtain and I made myself clear that I did not want to see anyone peeking!

Being Induced

With all three of my daughters, I did not get to experience what other women experience when they go into labor. What I mean is that I didn't experience contractions at home or count how much time there was between contractions while pacing around my living room. This is because I was induced for all three deliveries. My first daughter was born when I was forty-one weeks' pregnant, my second daughter was born at forty weeks and four days, and for my third, I chose to be induced on forty weeks exactly as I know how my body loves holding babies hostage after forty weeks. When you are more than forty weeks' pregnant, the risks of stillbirth go up. The placenta is designed to last for only around forty weeks. After this time, it can start to fail, so the doctors like to induce you and get that baby out safely. Therefore, I have only ever experienced contractions after being induced.

When you're induced, the doctors give you an injection of oxytocin to get your contractions started. Apparently, this can cause them to be even stronger than in a normal labor. With my first daughter, it was insanely painful. I hadn't expected them to be that way because I read about them in books and they did not sound as bad. I don't know about you, but when I read something it often doesn't sound as bad as it is in reality. At the time, however, I was crying and asking for help. Now don't get me wrong, I know natural labor is crazy painful as well, and many women also cry in pain. I only know about my own experience. The other thing that made it hard is that I progressed so slowly. I think twelve hours passed during my first delivery, and I was only three centimeters dilated.

A slow labor is relatively common in first labors, so don't be too surprised if this happens to you. When I heard that was all I had achieved after so much pain for so long, I was so upset, I told them that's it, just do anything, give me an epidural, or give me a cesarean, just get me out of this misery! It was absolute agony. Luckily, they jumped into action with an epidural, and my pain was soon under control. It still took a long time for my first daughter to be delivered, but at least the agony was over.

Then the magical moment arrived: she was out. There are absolutely no words to describe the moment when someone holds up your child and you get to meet them. That moment when you see your child—the one you have felt wriggle, kick, and hiccup inside you for so many weeks—that moment is like nothing else. Congratulations!

Make It Hurt Less with Pain Relief

If you are giving birth at a government hospital here in the UAE, and you are having a normal delivery, the midwife is likely to be the main decision-maker about your pain relief. As much as you might want the doctor you have been seeing throughout the nine months of your pregnancy to be with you, there is a real chance he or she will be busy or unavailable. You will definitely not have that person there for the entire labor. Therefore, plan ahead if you would like to have a familiar face in the room and speak to your healthcare provider about your wishes. Make sure the doctor you are seeing is committed to be being there. Otherwise, the midwife will usually be in the room with you and will be the person who oversees your birth unless there is a problem. While it is possible to book a midwife to stay with you for the entire birth, this is not guaranteed as no one can predict when your contractions will start. The midwife's shift might end before you reach your next centimeter of dilation and another midwife on duty will come to assist.

It is important to have a midwife who is on your side. If you have strong opinions on pain relief or epidurals, put it in your birth plan and get your midwife on board. One of my friends' midwives told her she could not have an epidural because it was her first birth and she needed to feel the contractions to be able to push properly. Not helpful! The doctor who attended my second delivery also told me she was against epidural during the delivery. The pain was horrendous, and I would not have chosen her if I had known. *But just a side note: I love her so much and I am so glad that she was my doctor!* I understand now that it was my fault for not opening this subject with her beforehand!

What makes it worse is that for my second child, I had made sure to pick a doctor who would be with me, because I hadn't liked that the midwives didn't know me during my first delivery. It really worried me that the midwives only know what is written in your medical notes and nothing else.

During my second delivery the doctor, who I found out was against epidural right when the contractions started, only allowed me gas and air, which is supposed to make it better but it did not do it for me. It was actually horrendous. I had to survive a second induced labor on basically no pain relief.

Whether you normally like to control things or like to go with the flow, you should always create a birth plan before the big day and discuss it with your obstetrician, especially if epidural and pain management are important to you. Write all your ideas and views down and show them what you want to happen. Do you want an epidural? Do you want monitoring or not? Monitoring can be useful, but it also means you have to lie on a bed and not move around. Many women find it more comfortable to stand for a lot of their labor. Do you want a water birth or a birthing ball? All these things should be considered and discussed before you start feeling those contractions. Of course, you may throw away your plan and change your mind when it actually happens. But if you want something and find out that you can't have it, like I did, that can be really stressful.

All About Epidurals and Other Forms of Pain Relief

Epidurals must be given early enough in the labor to be effective. The anesthetist puts a needle in near your spine. Contractions come very close together near the end—just seconds apart—so it makes giving an epidural impossible. So if epidural is what you definitely want, make sure to get to the hospital as soon as the contractions begin. Of course, the contractions are also more painful near the end, so by the time you realize you want the epidural it may be too late.

There are other pain relief options if you decide you don't want an epidural or you aren't able to have one. Many women use Entonox (gas and air), just as my doctor gave me during my second child's delivery. A friend in the U.K. managed three days of labor on gas and air before finally needing more help, as she was so exhausted. She said it was painful, but the gas and air took the edge off the pain enough that she could cope with it.

Other women get relief from the pain through meditation and birthing pools. These are large, warm baths whose relaxing effect reduces stress and pain. Some women manage the entire delivery with a birthing pool and meditation. If you are experienced at meditating, it is worth considering.

But like most women nowadays, you will probably want the epidural, because they really work. The main drawback is that they paralyze you from the injection point downwards for hours and hours. So you will be unable to stand up or walk about once you have one. This seems worth it during the contractions, but once the baby is out it's not so great until the effect goes away. But the nurses do help a lot. In fact, they will even take your child off to the nursery so you can rest after the birth and don't have to start being a full-time parent straight away! I was able to get a night of sleep after my first daughter was born, which was a blessing.

New Dads

My husband was there for our children's deliveries and he was a wonderful support, although I did not allow him to see anything. Some women prefer their men to wait elsewhere and not see the actual birth, and I was definitely one of those. Birth is a messy business, so it is a personal choice. It is important to think about what you want on your delivery day so it goes well for you and your husband. While everyone focuses on the new mom, remember your husband has also just become a parent too.

I truly felt how sad it was when one of my friends told me how she went through most of her labor without her husband. He didn't arrive until half an hour before the delivery. As she had been refused an epidural, she was in complete agony by the time he walked in. She was squatting, she was crawling, she was moving around. Into this world of pain and contractions walked her husband, who asked her, "What's wrong?" I can only imagine her reply. She wanted to hit him with whatever was nearby. Some men can be so clueless. It's funny now, but it wasn't back then for her.

After you give birth, the umbilical cord needs to be cut. This connects the baby to the placenta. In the UAE it is typical for the father to cut the cord before he whispers the call to prayer in the baby's ear. Everything goes quiet, so this is the first thing they hear when they come into the world. This is such a special moment for the new dad. Saeed and I were so proud of our little girls, all 3.9kgs of our first one, all 3.4kgs of our second, and all 3.51 of the third.

You Still Have to Push After Your Baby Is Born!

Are you ready for this? Delivering the baby is not the end of the birth. You have worked so hard for so many hours, or even days, and now your baby is here all you want to do is rest and enjoy your child. Well, welcome to the new way of life for you. You want to do one thing, but you have a responsibility to do something else. It's called being a mom!

The first job that takes you away from what you want is delivering the placenta. You need to put the baby down and get this job done. If you've had an epidural, you might not know much about it. But if you haven't, you will have to push the placenta out like the baby, and it's hard work. Some people feel like they've had to deliver twins because the placenta can be very large and weigh more than the baby! But delivering the placenta quickly and well is important for your own safety. If it doesn't detach properly or any of it is left inside, the mother can hemorrhage. Don't worry, though: the midwives or your doctor know all about this and will guide you through it.

Going through that horrendous labor, especially my second one without pain relief, gave me huge respect for our ancestors. Thinking back to our parents and grandparents, I developed a major level of admiration for my mother and grandmother realizing they had survived all their labors this way with no pain relief other than traditional remedies, and at a very young age. Knowing my mother was married at twelve, and knowing what giving birth is like, I developed a lot of sympathy and empathy for what they went through. In the weeks after childbirth, you really start looking at women in a different way when you know they have children. It's like you are now part of a club that has survived a challenging experience!

The Hospital Reception

Ever since having my own children, I've wondered why it's only the child who gets presents on their birthday. Surely the mothers who work so hard and go through so much to get that person into the world deserve some recognition and thanks each year for their efforts! I think we should bring in a new tradition that moms are celebrated on their children's birthdays, complete with presents and treats! Sadly, the tradition seems to be that instead of being the center of attention, women are the planners and organizers of their children's birthdays. So much work every year! But the first one, the one when you meet your child for the first time, that is the big one. Here in the UAE and most Arab countries, it has become a well-organized party to which everyone is invited.

Once the placenta is out, you are truly exhausted but at least the pain is over. You will want to finally relax and get some rest, and you really deserve it. Thankfully, hospitals usually have nurseries, so you can have a bit of rest. But not for too long. New traditions have turned the birth into a party at the hospital, and it needs to be a good one. People will judge you on how well you do. You don't even get to wait until you get home to introduce the world to your baby because the world will come to you at the hospital. So get yourself cleaned up. It is time to be the hostess with the mostest.

Our experience of giving birth in this part of the world is different from some Western countries. Here, most of us have a private room and we stay in the hospital for a few days with the nursery watching the baby most of the time so we can rest, recover, and "entertain guests." We still have the large wards after the birth, often with three or four women in curtained bays, but we opt for the private rooms. When you are in a shared ward, you are encouraged to go home quickly to make room for the next person. If you are in a private room, they would want you to stay longer to pay more! Here we have developed a culture where the private room even becomes the venue for a whole event. It's like a reception and you are the host as you welcome friends and family to meet your new child. This reception has to be planned ahead of time with a full party-planning check list. You must have catering and nice flower arrangements with a theme and giveaways for your visitors. On top of this, the mommy is expected to wear something lacy or silky and appropriately lavish. There is a definite luxuriousness and style to the gown the woman wears when she greets the people who have come to see her and her child. It should be like a modest nightgown but very fancy, made from lace and silk. When I had my first daughter, I had a French designer make a few gowns for me. They were elegant, modest, almost regal, and completely UNCOMFORTABLE!

I asked my mother and my older sisters if they were expected to do all this when they had their kids, especially since my eldest sister had her first child back in 1995 when I was only 5 years old. They all confirmed that this is a new tradition that has developed more recently. Yes, people used to still come and visit at the hospital, but they did not expect to find much at the hospital room more than some homemade hot beverages in flasks and simple food brought in Tupperware or thermal food containers. It is part of a new culture that was formed in my generation and probably began around five to ten years ago. With my first pregnancy, I heard people asking me about my plans for the hospital reception. They wanted to know what I was going to do for the floral arrangement, what my theme was going to be, and so on. Honestly, I never thought that this should be something that I worry about ahead of time. It's hard enough to have a baby and think about everything you should do once this baby comes ahead of time, yet we still have the added pressure of creating a spectacular reception on top of that. I had to buy a lot of things from dinnerware to vases to giveaways! It was so much work when I already had a job and I kept wondering where would all this stuff go once I am discharged from the hospital. Instead, I found a woman who plans these events for a living. It was very expensive, but I didn't have the time or energy to do it myself and decided to just pay that sum of money and choose a theme that she has published on her Instagram page. It was a super classy theme with lots of lace, crystals, and she even brought her own French-style consoles to display the giveaways and food. All she had to do was change the colors from blue to pink.

When you hire a planner, everything must be ready a few weeks before your due date and all you have to do is ask somebody to inform the planner that you are in labor to start arranging everything in your private room.

After I had given birth and was rolled into my room on a hospital bed, I got a dreadful shock. It was nothing like we had discussed or what I had chosen. Everything was like a parody of what I had wanted. All the details were wrong and for some reason, there were pink Chinese paper lanterns hanging from the ceiling which I don't recall seeing on her Instagram page nor ordering in the first place. I was so angry. What made it worse was that I felt so hot. I was beginning to feel faint after the birth, and I was so overheated. I was sitting there fuming about how awful it was and getting hotter and hotter and the awful decorations made me feel worse. So I told my husband to call the planner and tell her to come immediately and take everything away. I didn't want my guests to see this.

To replace the missing arrangements, I called my friend's flower shop and asked them to send over a few beautiful pink flower arrangements. Then I sent my husband to the mall to buy things like table covers and accessories. It's funny now, but the poor man was running around the shops instead of looking at his newborn child because of the room arrangement disaster. If I could go back, I would just let that entire thing slide. It is ridiculous how society makes us care about materialistic things instead of the stuff that matters—that baby, that miracle!

For my second delivery, I decided to do things a little differently. I had been so uncomfortable in what I was wearing for my first delivery, so this time I wore cotton pajamas with lacy details. I wasn't going to suffer again, add pressure to pressure, and feel uncomfortable. So I bought cotton fabric, some lace, and I designed pant pajamas and asked a tailor to sew them for me. I was very comfortable in them, and I would recommend this for every delivery. I would never wear extravagant gowns ever again.

Since we are expected to have this reception event, although I believe it is a little ridiculous, I did everything myself for my second child. I bought the vases, the dinner set, the table cloths, everything. I labelled them in boxes so my in-laws and my husband would know how to arrange everything in my room and when the guests arrived, it would be all ready. To avoid the issue of storing all those things, I basically distributed them to my sister and other people in my family. Problem solved.

My plan for when I have a third child was to try to make the most out of this hospital reception and book a photographer for a little family photoshoot at the room. It just feels like such a waste to spend so much time, effort, and money to decorate and not have a keepsake. However, my hospital experience with my third child was completely different, thanks to the COVID-19 outbreak. Visitors were not allowed in and I only had my husband with me. That peace and quiet at the hospital for two days gave me a lot of time to bond with my new baby, an experience that was extremely different than my earlier deliveries. An experience I totally loved!

After my labor, all three times, it's an understatement to say I felt exhausted. I don't remember much from this time actually because I was so tired. One thing I do know is that if you can have a private room after your delivery, I highly recommend it. It makes such a difference to have extra time, space, and privacy as you get to know your child.

With my first daughter I remember the room being very hot. I was asking for AC and for water. They told me they couldn't turn the AC on because of the baby. It felt so hot to me, but no one else seemed to think it was bad. It turns out I was feeling faint. Feeling hot is one of the things that can happen before you pass out. I felt like I was standing outside in the sun in 50-degree weather. I remember that vividly. I lost consciousness and everyone thought that it was from blood loss. Later on, they told me that my blood pressure had gone down. The hospital staff acted quickly, tilting the bed up so the blood would flow to my head. Bizarrely, I remember that. I know I wasn't completely conscious, but I wasn't all the way out, either. The next thing I remember is opening my eyes and seeing my husband with tears in his eyes. He thought he had lost me. And his whole life flashed before his eyes—poor guy!

Luckily, their little bed trick sorted it out and I was given some iron tablets to take at home. That night they took the baby to the nursery and let me rest. I really needed it. The next day the nurse came and said she was going to help me take a shower. You are generally very sore and uncomfortable after giving birth, and your body doesn't just snap back to its old shape and energy! You know how your muscles feel the day after you do some weights at the gym or an extra-long workout? Well, your abdominal muscles just did the equivalent of a marathon without any training. Everything is going to hurt, and having someone help you shower is totally necessary!

What Not to Wear

While most of your thoughts are all about your new baby, you still have some room in your head to notice what's happening to you. Let's talk about your belly for a minute. The day after I gave birth to my first daughter, I looked down and I thought I was still pregnant. I didn't expect to have such a big tummy after giving birth. For some reason, I thought my body would snap back into shape and I would be completely fit again all of a sudden. I'm sorry to be the one to break the news to you if that's what you're expecting, too, but that just doesn't happen. Your body was stretched so big, you couldn't see your toes. Your belly isn't going to fit into your pre-pregnancy clothes again for a long, long time. The one time I was ever with someone giving birth (and I don't think I would want to repeat that experience ever again) was with my niece. Right after her baby was born, the first question she asked the nurses while still gasping for air was "how much weight did I lose?" She truly cracked me up.

In your hospital bag, pack some big knickers and very loose comfortable clothes to wear after the birth, especially once the guests are gone. You want something that you can easily move out of the way or even take off when you're learning to breastfeed. You might even want to buy a new maternity outfit just for after the birth, so it fits comfortably and so that you can feel like you've got a treat waiting for you! Just make sure not to get over-excited and purchase your size prior to getting pregnant.

You're Still Contracting, Honey!

Now we've got that little shocker out of the way, I've got more news for you. Your contractions aren't quite over yet. No, I'm serious. Your womb is going to contract down to its pre-pregnant size over the next few weeks, and some of those contractions can HURT. Some people might just get a little stomachache, but some of those contractions can be eye-watering. And while we're sharing icky bits, you're going to have the period from hell. Get in a massive stack of the biggest maternity pads you can find, as you will need them. Plus, after giving birth, going to the toilet can feel like your womb is about to be born, too, unless you've been stitched up—which is fashionable in this part of the world right now. Then there is coughing and sneezing. That definitely makes you feel like your rear end is going to fall out. These are the icky reality bits they don't tell us about. I wonder why!

How Times Change

There is something very grounding to realize that my mother went through the same things I did when she had me in 1990. But large parts of her experience were different from mine. There were still ten years left of the twentieth century, and the world was a very different place. The United Arab Emirates was still less than a quarter of a century old. The giant metropolis of Abu Dhabi and the city of Dubai with its famous man-made islands were only beginning to emerge from the landscape, enormous cranes dotted the skyline, and I was a very unexpected late surprise for my parents.

My closest sibling, my brother Rashed, is six years older than me, and my mom had already decided to stop having babies when I came along due to being diabetic. We have had some very honest conversations about how my mother felt about having an eighth child, especially since I became a mother myself. Eight is almost an average number of children for women in my mother's generation, partly because they started families younger than we do today. Some women would have ten or more children, just like large Catholic families did back then.

My mother was a child when she had her first baby and was in her late thirties when she had me. She was upset to know that she was expecting a child six year after having my brother, but she knew I was a gift from God, and who was she to refuse? The trouble was that she had Type 1 diabetes. It was a very difficult pregnancy and she had seven other kids to care for, of whom the oldest was already twenty and the youngest was six. Managing a home with so many children would be exhausting for anybody, let alone a diabetic with all the exhaustion that comes with pregnancy.

It's situations like this where the Gulf style of living together with extended family can be a great strength. My mother ended up spending most of her pregnancy in hospital while my older sisters helped run the home for the rest of us.

Just as it was for me when I was on bed rest with a broken leg, lying in bed all day was hard on my mother. I think she, too, was frustrated to be so still—she's an energetic, active woman usually—but she also felt sick. By the time I arrived, she was more than happy for me to be out! Although she may have been upset with this pregnancy, that feeling disappeared and she loved me. I was her eighth birth, so the delivery went pretty much as expected with no new surprises! After a few deliveries, your body knows what to do, so it just gets on with it. For the other births my father would usually drop her at the hospital to give birth and drive back to stay with my siblings. Then the hospital would call him when the baby was born, so they would all come to the hospital to meet the new addition to the family.

I love modern Emirati life, but when I heard what my mother told me about having children in the old days, it did make me wonder if we have lost a little something of ourselves. She told me, "Every period of time has its own flavor. Back then, life was not as easy as it is nowadays. However, what was better was the fact that everyone was there to help you. The neighbors would help if your family were not there to help. There was a sense of community and close ties that made everyone feel like family. Nowadays, everything is easy, but people have grown far apart, which is sad. Everything a woman needs nowadays can be bought with money, while back then people were ready to jump up and help even if the person did not ask for it."

Giving Birth in the Old Days

My mother comes from a Bedouin background; she lived in the desert her whole life until the country was established and the cities began to grow. My mother gave birth to her first child in 1970 at Sara Hosman Hospital, which was referred to as "Elamreekeya." This stood for "The American" back then. The American was the first maternity hospital in Sharjah. It opened in 1951 and closed down in the 1990s. It was then turned into a historical place that is open for the public to visit. Most of my siblings were born there, but I was born at Dubai Hospital.

Before the hospitals, women gave birth at home. There wasn't any other option. Generally, women used to deliver by holding a stick placed vertically in the ground. They would squat while holding that stick and deliver in that position. The woman's mother or a neighbor would assist the birth, unless there was a midwife living nearby. Of course, when I say *midwife,* I mean a woman with experience assisting with births. They obviously did not have degrees back then. There would usually be somebody rubbing the woman's back to help her deliver the baby, which could be her mother or her neighbor. Sometimes, if a woman lived with her husband away from their family, the husband would even assist her in delivering the child.

Pain relief is obviously a big issue when you're trying to push something the size of a melon out of your body. But back in the day, all they had was a laxative-like herbal mixture, which helped in inducing labor. This was called "*hlool*" and it contained castor, coriander seeds, acacia, wild thyme, fennel, and fenugreek. It had the same effect as castor oil. No pain relief at all.

If that doesn't sound terrible enough, I asked my mother what people used to do if something went wrong. What if the baby was in the wrong position? I almost wished I hadn't asked. She told me that if something was wrong with the position of the baby, the woman would be placed in the middle of a blanket or a large piece of cloth. Her husband and brothers or whoever was around to help would then hold the four edges of that blanket and keep shaking the woman until she started screaming. They would then let her get off that blanket and get into position to deliver. Now that we have surgical theaters and C-sections, this seems so strange. But if the baby was stuck, you can understand they would try anything to make it move or both the mother and baby could die. Of course, there are situations this wouldn't help, and many more women died in childbirth than now. We are blessed to have modern facilities.

In those days, my mother told me that after a woman gave birth, whoever attended her delivery would cut the umbilical cord by first squeezing it and pushing the fluid/blood that is in it back to the placenta, then measuring three fingers away from the newborn and cutting it using a razor. They would then tie it and leave it to heal and fall off. The placenta was then buried under the ground. We're not sure why that was done, but it was the tradition.

Once a woman survives the birth, my mother says, an old ritual was performed that was supposed to help her recover. This ritual included sand with camel's urine on it, mixed with hot sand taken from under a campfire. This mixture would be spread on the ground and the woman would be asked to lie down on it on her back. Her stomach would be wrapped tightly with a piece of cloth and she would be covered with blankets. The heat under her back was supposed to help her relax her muscles. Talking with my mother, we are not sure what the supposed benefits of the camel urine were, but that is what used to be done. The woman would then sleep until the next day and would wake up feeling energetic and ready to take care of her child.

As I said, the womb shrinks down over the weeks after birth, and this can be quite painful for some women. Back before cities and hospitals, a method that was used to flatten the woman's stomach after birth was to place a big warm rock on it for some time every day for forty days after delivery. This helped the uterus shrink and people believed it prevented a saggy stomach. Some people still do that up to this day!

Another area rife with tradition for postpartum women was the special food they had to eat. After giving birth, the woman was advised to eat a very high calorie diet of white rice, ghee, and liver. This was usually prepared by whoever was taking care of her, whether that was her mother, her neighbor, or her in-laws. Scientifically, there is a lot to be said for this tradition. Women often lose a lot of blood during labor, so the liver would help replenish her iron. And she would need energy: the carbohydrates in white rice and the fats in ghee would all help her recover her strength. But the woman was also given eggshells to eat. This is supposed to be a good source of calcium, which is diminished during pregnancy when our bodies will even take it from our own bones to support our growing child if we do not eat enough of it, but it sounds rather crunchy and not very appetizing! This diet had to be followed for seven days after the birth. The mind-boggling thing is that the people who came up with these traditions were completely uneducated. One must wonder: how did they come up with all of that?

Women were also given what is called *hrairowa*. This is a drink that sounds suspiciously miraculous. It was said to strengthen her, give her back her energy, help with milk supply, and flatten the stomach. Now that's the kind of tradition I like the sound of! *Hrairowa* is a mixture of many different things, but the main ingredients are garden cress seeds, black pepper, and flour. I am not sure about the scientific basis for those claims but I find it delicious!

Tradition Vs. Science

The traditions of our cultures developed for a reason. But there are some rather dubious claims people make about what women should do to get healthy again after having a child. For example, my mom always insisted we should wear a wrap like a corset around the stomach, so our tummy would go back. It seemed reasonable, and I tried very hard to do this as I wanted to regain my old body shape. But at the same time, I was trying to breastfeed. At a breastfeeding class, I learned that the corset would not help the milk supply. So, because I was really eager to breastfeed, I ditched the corset. It made me think, though. The pressure on women to lose the baby weight is definitely greater than it was before. More so than the pressure of breastfeeding! Social media, like Instagram and all the celebrities who lose the baby weight immediately after giving birth, make things very hard for us. They are doing photoshoots and sometimes use Photoshop, which really puts unhelpful pressure on us.

I listened to the scientific advice in my books, and waited until six weeks had passed before I tried to work out. I hired a personal trainer and started to work out regularly. But it was difficult for me to get back to the shape I was before getting pregnant, and even now, three deliveries later, I still carry some extra weight. Having a baby changes our bodies more than we realize. Our feet get bigger and spread, our breasts change size because of milk supply. Even our hands change! Looking at my own hands, I realized how, after all the water retention disappeared and my fingers returned to normal size, there is extra skin that makes me feel wrinkly!

We punish ourselves while trying to return to the body of a childless woman, but it's normal to develop a new body shape once you're a mom. Maybe we should embrace that idea a little more, and give ourselves a break! Our bodies have undergone major changes to bring a life to life, yet we want it to go back to the shape it was before undergoing the most amazing thing a woman's body can ever do? Self-acceptance and self-love are what we should embrace.

Chapter 5
You Have a Baby, Now What?

After the delivery, for all the time you're still at the hospital, you're kind of in a protected cocoon. There are nurses and other people around who will take the baby away to the nursery so you can rest, and when the baby is around, they will help you learn how to latch your baby on to breastfeed, how to put on a diaper, and so on. But they can't hold your hand forever. There comes a time when you have to go home and start figuring out parenting all on your own.

You may well feel like you've done the hard part, but the birth really is just the beginning. Now you have a teeny tiny real-life little person who needs you for absolutely everything twenty-four hours a day. Nobody is ever fully prepared for that. It is almost always a shock to the system. While you are pregnant, you are exhausted but you can try to sleep when you need it. When your baby has arrived, you must get up and work out what is wrong whenever he or she needs you, even if that is two minutes after your own eyes closed or when you are on the toilet, in the shower, or just made a hot meal. Your needs become completely secondary to theirs. It doesn't help that newborn babies literally don't know how to do anything. It can be a little amusing to see the shock on their faces when they poop, but you will need to teach them the ways of their bodies and of the world, and help them feel safe and secure. It's a big responsibility.

Just like most moms, a friend of mine found it very hard to adjust her sleeping with her baby's. She is an early riser, so she goes to sleep early, but her son was the complete opposite. She hadn't expected that it would be hard to find a routine that worked for them both, especially since she raised her little brother and two of her cousins herself. But there is a world of difference between helping out a mom during the day and being the mom yourself.

Another unexpected problem she faced was the sheer number of visitors she had to entertain, just like many new moms these days in the UAE. In our culture, we do a lot of entertaining and spending time with our extended families. People always love to meet new babies, and visitors want to meet the new member of the family as soon as possible. But the exhausted, sleepless mother, who is trying to learn how to care for her baby, is also expected to host the guests and be welcoming. The truth is the new mom just wants everyone to either go away, or bring her drinks and snacks, not the other way around! For my friend, it was even harder because her sister and cousin both delivered within a month of her delivery but had to return to work and university, so she ended up being the main carer for all three infants during the day. The rounds of feeding, diaper changes, and soothing were relentless. Then, on top of that, she had to entertain. It was too much really, but she survived.

Another friend of mine had a completely different experience. For her, having her first child was amazing. She told me, "It felt unbelievable that this human wasn't in my life just a month ago and now here we are." What made the difference was that her family helped a lot. The nonstop crying, no sleeping, and lack of showers was very hard. Like every new parent, what surprised her most was how her child could stay awake for so long. She had been told that babies should sleep at least eighteen hours, but hers slept for eight hours at the most. What no one had told her was that babies sleep for short amounts in between being awake. They do sleep for eighteen hours, but not in one go! She was lucky to get a baby who slept for a solid eight hours.

Going Home with Your Child

The first challenge of parenting is getting home. Don't laugh. I can see you raising your eyebrows. Because, of course, you have driven many times. But with your new baby in the car, it isn't as easy as it sounds.

Did you know that some hospitals wouldn't allow you to leave the hospital before ensuring that a baby car seat is installed in your car? The hospital where I delivered my first child did not let me walk out of the door until they made sure the baby was safely strapped into an infant car seat. You definitely should not cradle your baby in your arms as you leave even if no one told you that you must have a car seat. Your number one priority as a mother now is to keep your child safe, and a car seat is just the most important item of your trip home. I love how when I delivered Shereena, the hospital gave us a car seat to take her home in; it was a very nice gesture.

Going home with our new baby for the first time, it was just the three of us in the car. We had gone from being a couple who drives around in a coupe to being a family in an SUV, and it felt like a milestone in our life together. I remember my husband driving incredibly slowly. He was so stressed about having the baby in the car. He thought he was driving very carefully, but actually it was much too slow. It was crazy how he would take a turn—like in slow motion—him, the racing fanatic! I mean I know there is a baby in the car, but you don't have to do that!

Make sure you watch a few videos on YouTube on how to use the infant's car seat belt and how to tighten it the right way so the baby is strapped in safely. Some babies actually suffocate in car seats because the strap is too tight. If it is loose, the baby's head can drop down and it can stop breathing. Newborn babies do not have the strength in their necks to lift their own heads. And never let them sleep in a car seat without being properly strapped for the same reason. Of course, this doesn't happen to most people, but you have to know all the precautions.

After you have a baby, your body needs to switch back to being a nonpregnant body. You are no longer growing a little life inside you, but you will start producing milk to feed your baby and your uterus needs to shrink back to its pre-pregnancy size. Pregnant women usually retain a lot of water near the end of the pregnancy, and this all needs to be shed. It can be a good idea to sleep with towels under you for a few weeks, as you'll have night sweats. And, if you're not feeling awful enough, you will lose a lot of hair. When you're pregnant you stop losing hair, so it becomes thicker and shinier, which is wonderful. But once the baby is out, all that extra hair starts falling out. It can be terrifying to see handfuls of it disappear down the drain in the shower. This is perfectly normal, so try not to worry. The other big change to your body is all the different hormones that are starting or stopping in the days and weeks after labor. This can really affect your emotions and it's something that really affected me personally. I had to find ways to help myself recover.

The Baby Blues

Traditionally in this culture, after a woman gives birth, she is not allowed to leave the house for forty days—not even to attend weddings or visit women who just got married or go to mourning. They say the reason is that if she were to get a very bad case of fever, she might die or her child might die. But this is just a myth. It's something they used to believe in. I heard that some families still think this is true. Fortunately, I wasn't prevented from leaving the house. It was fine. And thank goodness, because I was badly affected by the baby blues and I believe it would have gotten much worse if I had been cooped up at home for so long.

Please don't be dismissive of yourself if you start to feel down after the baby arrives. Nobody starts off knowing how to parent. We are all learning as we go along, and I have realized this is probably true for the whole time your children live with you. I didn't know how to teach someone to eat before I had a child, but now I do. I have never had a teenager, so I don't know how to parent one yet. Though I am sure that when I am faced with a hormonal teenager, I will learn and do my best when I get there!

It's no surprise that many women develop baby blues, or postpartum depression. With my first one, it was really overwhelming and I was crying the whole time. I was so dramatic. But making it worse was the feeling that I wasn't able to do anything with her. I got overwhelmed and had thoughts that my baby could die at any minute. My husband was going to go to the army soon after she was born, which probably made things worse. When I had my second baby, I had these blues again but not as severely.

When I look back at that time, I can see that another reason was my confusion over what I had read and what I was being told. For instance, I read that babies should not be given water, as it interferes with their body's ability to absorb nutrients from breastmilk and formula. The books said their kidneys cannot process excess fluid before six months of age. In my culture, though, babies are given water all the time, and it is considered inhumane to ban them from it because milk makes them thirsty! I wasn't sure what to believe. These contradictions are difficult to work out when you're trying to do the best for your child and cope with interrupted sleep. I was constantly feeling ashamed for believing things I read which, as a new mom, made me feel confused, scared, incapable, and really, really down.

I ended up deciding that the book advice was inapplicable because those countries were in low temperate regions. They didn't need to worry about how hot the weather is in the UAE, where dehydration is a constant, real threat for babies. This is a good example of using your own intelligence and applying the advice that works for you in your situation. I decided that sometimes my baby might need a drink other than milk. If you know your baby has had the milk that is recommended for their age and weight, there is no harm in giving them a top-up of clean, fresh sterilized water in a syringe or bottle. It was when I started developing some confidence in caring for my baby that the blues lifted. I realized that I was doing okay and she was fine.

Becoming a parent for the first time is very hard. But for women, hormones can make it harder if they are one of the unfortunate ones to get the baby blues. Postpartum depression can be as mild as feeling a bit low and crying more easily at things, or as serious as making the mom feel suicidal. Sometimes, it can be so serious that the mother thinks she is a danger to her child, and it can cause her to reject the baby. Thankfully, this situation is extremely rare. But if you start to feel as if you can't cope, it is really important to tell your family and your physician. There are many ways new moms can get help with these powerful feelings, and it is nothing to be ashamed of. Would you be ashamed if you broke a leg? Would you struggle on without getting treatment? Would you try to do things that are impossible with a broken leg and keep that broken leg hidden? The answer is definitely no. Then do not be ashamed if your hormones are affecting you too much and you need some help. That is what doctors are for.

When it was especially bad, I found myself calling my best friend, Noura, and crying. She used to ask me, "Why are you crying?" and I had to reply that I really didn't know. It felt so strange to be crying and not be able to control it. I didn't want to cry, and feeling that I was out of control about it made me cry even more! The instant anyone would mention breastfeeding; I would start sobbing because I could not breastfeed. I felt like I was depriving my child from one of her rights. But now that I think about it, why do people ask if you breastfeed or not? Why should this be a topic to discuss and make the mother feel worse than she already does? I know that my emotional rollercoaster was caused by hormones, but people's intrusion on what you are or not doing as a mom does not make it go away and doesn't make you feel better. If anything, it adds more pressure to the extent that you want to scream. It did help to call my friend and to let my husband know about my feelings though. Finding support from your friends and family can start to help you recover.

Usually when Emirati women give birth, they go to their parents' home instead of the marital home for forty days after the birth. There, they have the support of their own mother, who can teach them about how to care for the baby, and the idea is that they can recover from the birth without their husband seeing them go through it. But that isn't how it happened for me. I went back home with my husband, and my mother was in another city. The help people were offering didn't always feel like help, either. It was important for me to parent my child the way I had learned how to from the modern-day books. I had clear ideas about how I wanted to care for her, and I really didn't want to feel like someone was there bossing me around. People can mean well, but if they interfere too much it can make the new mom feel worse!

That's why I tried not to be close to people who felt like they could tell me what to do, or try to force me to do something I was not comfortable with.

Breastfeeding: Just Stick Your Baby on Your Boob

All baby routines are centered on two things: eating and sleeping. When you have your baby, the nurses and midwives at the hospital help you start to breastfeed. They show you how to get the baby to latch on and how to burp it afterwards. The milk you make in the first few days is a special kind called colostrum. This has all sorts of amazing health benefits in it for your baby. Despite all their help, truthfully, even though they'd shown me how to feed her a few times, I didn't really know what to do. There is such a difference between seeing it on a video and trying it yourself with a real live baby. But I was trying my hardest to make it work and I was becoming very frustrated.

One thing the midwives insisted on was not to give her a bottle at home. They told me this because they believed that if I did, it would give her "nipple confusion." Nipple confusion is a big deal for midwives and they assured me it won't let her latch onto my nipple. So that meant we couldn't use bottles at all. I took their advice very seriously, because I really wanted to get this right. I had always known I was going to breastfeed, so it was a real shock that no matter what I tried, she wasn't latching. I asked for help every time I fed her at the hospital, but they brushed me off and simply told me to keep trying. It was so hard. Hearing your child cry from hunger is utterly heartbreaking. When you are in the hospital, their solution is for you to give milk through a syringe. I did that and she was still crying the whole time. I'm sure she felt like she was being starved.

I had always known I would breastfeed my babies, and I had planned to do it for two years for each child. I think this is healthy. But it felt like I was failing. As much as she cried and screamed because she was hungry, I couldn't seem to get her to feed from me. So a few days after leaving the hospital, I went back to get some help. They tried again to show me how to latch her on, but one of the nurses told me that I had flat nipples and that was why I had problems. I had never heard of that. I thought nipples were just nipples. How could there be different types? I then learned that there are inverted nipples and flat nipples, as well as the usual ones that stick outwards. I was told it was not impossible to breastfeed with flat nipples, but it would be harder. I felt so disappointed. I had been so sure breastfeeding would be easy, and I felt like my body had let me down. It definitely contributed to my low mood.

For me, flat nipples meant breastfeeding would not work. Period. I determinedly continued to try to breastfeed, but it felt like the baby's crying became continuous. I even tried to express the milk using a breast pump. After hours and hours of the screams of our distressed daughter, eventually my husband had enough. He said, "That's IT! I don't care whether she latches or not. The baby's hungry—just give her a bottle." It was a relief in a way. Of course, I hadn't planned to bottle-feed, so we didn't have any of the things we needed, but she was going to be fed soon.

I sent Saeed out to buy a bottle, bottle sterilizer, and all the paraphernalia of bottle feeding.

We rushed around opening the boxes, reading the instructions, and trying to sterilize things and prepare the milk at breakneck speed—all with baby screams in the background. It was like someone had sped up a film. But I will never forget the moment we gave her that first bottle. The minute she drank, she raised her tiny little legs right up as if she were drinking with her entire body. It's like she was saying FINALLY. You could see the change come over her almost as if she were resurrected!

That night we found the answer for our family. But I was sad about it for a long time. It wasn't how I had seen myself as a mother. I had always thought I would be one of those moms who just whipped her breast out any time her child was hungry. I never considered that I might not be able to do it. The books and videos made it seem so simple. So did the staff at the hospital. But breastfeeding can be hard. If you think about it, both you and your baby are novices at this. You're learning together—the blind leading the blind—and unless you have really great support, it could be upsetting and stressful even if you do eventually get there. For a long while, I wondered whether, if my mother had been with me, maybe I could have done it. I did feel like a failure and that hurt me. But I wasn't a failure at all.

Bottle feeding wasn't part of the image I had created for myself. But looking back, I can see it was the right choice for us. Bottle feeding isn't for everyone, but don't let anyone make you feel bad if you discover it's what your family needs. It feels very wrong that we are made to feel ashamed for something we cannot control. I did not design my breast. It is the way it is. Some women simply can't produce enough milk; some babies can't latch; there are many reasons why a mother and baby might not be able to learn to feed together. And I feel society should support them instead of judging them.

Once we had agreed we were going to feed our baby with formula, things became much less stressful and everyone was happier, especially our daughter. Midwives and nurses don't like to talk about formula as an option, but this puts unfair pressure on moms who are having a tough time with it. Because of the baby blues, life with a bottle still wasn't perfect, but it was much better.

One of the girls I know found breastfeeding hard. Like me, she wanted to breastfeed her baby exclusively. But she felt judged, too. People around her told her that breast milk isn't enough at nighttime, and that is why the baby wasn't sleeping for very long. She was pressured by the idea that formula would make the baby sleep longer. Everyone who visited her had some advice of their own about what to do after having a baby. She found it was all confusing. For example, her cousin told her not to drink water, as it would make her have a belly. She listened and ended up feeling dehydrated. Now, when she thinks about it, she can see it was a ridiculous thing to say. We need water in order to increase milk supply. But her exhausted brain just couldn't find the arguments when she was learning how to cope with her first child. She feels she learned a lot from her first child experience and this gave her confidence to do things her own way for her other children. She still feels guilty that she only breastfed her first baby for two months due to the pressure, when she managed to exclusively breastfeed her second and third child for six months each.

I spoke to older women in my family about how babies were fed in the past. I couldn't believe that my problem was not something completely new. What did women do before formula? I discovered that after the birth and the umbilical cord was cut, the baby used to be wrapped and left until the mother had been taken care of. During the first three days, it was believed that the mother could not breastfeed, so one of the neighbors or her sister would breastfeed the child until she could do it herself. Now we know that the tiny amounts of milk produced in those first days are just different from the main milk supply that comes in around day three. Colostrum has essential nutrients that are really important for newborn babies. But the Bedouin tradition meant the baby got both colostrum and a full stomach in those vulnerable early days. Because of my own situation, I love that if the mother couldn't breastfeed at all, the neighbors would have continued breastfeeding the child until he or she is six months old, after which the baby would start to be given goat's milk. The family and the community was there, ready to help. Sometimes though, if there isn't anyone available to breastfeed the child, I was told that goat's milk would be given directly once the child is born. My mother added, "Since bottles were not available back then, they used to use any glass bottle that was available – be it oil bottle or jasmine extract bottle. They would wash the bottle, then use the leather from any mammal to create the teat. This is usually made using the leather or the skin from the mammal's paw because it is soft. This piece would be wrapped around the neck of the bottle and they would create an opening in the middle to encourage milk flow."

For me, bottle feeding was definitely the right solution for all three of my children. I would say though that if you can breastfeed and you don't have any issues in terms of breastfeeding or having baby latch, please do it. It's much better for the baby in many, many, many ways than formula. Some people have this perception that formula has all of these vitamins and these minerals, and there's no way that our breast milk could have all of these. They think, "I have deficiencies myself so how can my milk be good for the baby?" All of this is nonsense. Your breastmilk is the perfect food for your infant. You don't want to believe propaganda from companies who want to make money selling you formula. If the baby needs any extra supplements, the doctor will tell you. For me, I felt like I wanted that closeness with the baby. Even though I know it's almost the same when you hold the baby and a bottle, I do feel like I missed out and it is something I was deprived of.

Since I couldn't breastfeed, I gave my children formula up until the age of one, then I switched to camel milk. Camel milk is now seen as more beneficial than cow's milk. It was hard for me to find fresh camel's milk for my children on our travels, because not many places outside the Gulf have camels, except in zoos. During that time, my daughters drank full-fat fresh cow's milk when we were overseas. That was the case until powdered camel milk sachets became available in the market!

Things Are Going to Get Messy

Just when you think you've got your baby in a good feeding and sleeping routine, they reach the age when they start to need more than milk. Weaning is something else everybody has an opinion on. Everyone thinks they know best about what age your baby should start solids, what kind of food they should start with, and how they should eat it.

It's good to hear everyone's opinions, but at the end of the day, it is your child and you know them better than anyone. You will know what the right time is for your baby to wean. I began weaning at five months for all three of my daughters, simply because some people recommended weaning at four months, while other people said I had to wait until six months for solid food. So I decided to pick a point in the middle and the pediatrician agreed with me.

My mother gave me some great advice about finding the right time. There are signs we can look out for. These include babies starting to suck their hands. This shows they are hungry. If they are starting to suck their hands more than fifteen to thirty minutes before their next feeding is due, then they might be ready for solid food. They will also start to be interested in your food and watching you eat. They may even try to grab your food. That's a pretty strong sign. One important part of weaning is that babies need to be able to sit up by themselves before they are ready to eat solids. This is because of the risk of choking and the development of their ability to swallow well. If they can sit upright in a high chair unsupported and pick up toys from the tray to put in their mouths, they are ready to begin solid food.

Feeding babies is a messy business, no matter which way you do it. You will quickly learn that food with tomato wrecks baby clothes, for example. The stain never comes out! Also, some babies have very independent personalities. They can reject the food completely because they feel frustrated about not holding the spoon themselves. You will want to bathe your baby after every meal at some points! Some moms can't cope with that level of mess, but it is good to let the baby have that control. You don't want them to develop issues around food. One trick to get around this is to have two spoons for every meal. One is for the baby to hold and stick in her own mouth; the other is the one you use to quickly pop food in between the baby's own attempts.

Baby-led weaning is a fashion in some parts of Europe and America. This is a feeding technique that helps babies become independent eaters. These babies are not given pureed food or fed by a spoon by their parents. The idea is that purees were not available in the past and are kind of unnatural. In baby-led weaning, there are no jars or packets. Everything the baby eats is the same as you would eat yourself. You may even move some food from your plate to the baby's plate, so they can see it is the same as Mommy's. At the start the baby will just suck the food they are holding, or they will have a fist of mashed potato. Most of it will end up on the floor and in their hair. But eventually, they will learn to put it in their mouth and to use the spoon themselves.

If the food you want to give your baby can be mashed with a spoon, it is okay to give a baby who is just starting to wean. If it won't mash, or if it won't disintegrate when they suck it, then it is not suitable. For example, you wouldn't give a baby chicken as one of their first foods. You also wouldn't give babies food that can block their windpipe, like peas or grapes. I used a great baby feeder to help my babies have control and feed themselves. It helped reduce the risk of choking and allowed them to explore different flavors safely—and less messily! The chunky handle was perfect for a baby to grasp, while the mesh pocket could hold all sorts of food, like chunks of banana or cooked apple. It was a safety device that really worked for my family. Just search for the newest baby feeder available and read the reviews for assurance of quality.

Simple safety rules for peas, grapes, and so on are important to remember. If it is round and small enough to swallow whole like a grape, cut it in half lengthways so it cannot block their windpipe. If it is very small and round like a pea, wait until they have learned the pincer grip (using thumb and forefinger) before giving it to them. They will love to pick it up and feed themselves. If they have developed the pincer grip, they will also have developed enough control of their tongue and mouth to manage more difficult foods like this.

There are some great resources to help you know what foods babies can have at different stages of weaning. I found a wonderful chart on Pinterest that listed the foods from four months to fully weaned, and I stuck to it for all three daughters. Just search online for "baby feeding chart" and many will come up. We started with simply baby rice cereal, as babies can't take strong flavors at first. Simple, plain tastes that are not too sweet or too anything is the key. Once they have learned to swallow this safely, they can move on to try more flavors and thicker textures until they can try to chew.

Cutting food into stick shapes that the baby can hold will allow them to try things independently. Cooked carrot sticks, sweet potato, pieces of dry toast, and so on work well this way. Babies also like these because a harder piece of food can help with teething. But sometimes a bit can break off and a baby can gag on it. This is terrifying. But the baby's gag reaction is always there and it will protect them. What you mustn't do is overreact or you risk giving them an aversion to that food. Try to sit on your hands for a moment to see if they can gag the food back out. If they manage it themselves, which they will in 99.9 percent of cases, they learn they can cope and they won't be scared. If you jump up and shout and slap them on the back, they will become frightened as they see that you are frightened. This could put them off that food or even off eating for a while. So do your best to be reassuring and sound calm when a baby gags. But of course, learn baby first aid and what to do in case of real choking. This is something every parent should know about.

While it is empowering and fun to let babies feed themselves, sometimes you just need the convenience of a jar or pouch of baby food. My life was often too hectic to let my babies feed themselves at home. I would usually need to be out all day going from city to city, shopping or visiting people and, of course, the babies would have to come, too. I travel a lot, so premade baby food was a life-saver. I would tie a large bib around her neck and feed her in the stroller, which is like a convenient high chair. A few wipes and the baby is usually clean again, though it is surprising how often they manage to get food in their hair!

These days, it is important to give your baby organic food and try to find ones that are free from genetically modified ingredients. In the past, the important thing was that the food had a good range of fruit and vegetables in it. People didn't know about organic or GM. It wasn't an issue. I've heard that some moms now put their children on the paleo diet, but this seems extreme. It's just a fad. The important thing is feeding your baby natural food that gives a wide range of nutrients to help the child grow.

What Color Is That?!

The world of baby poop is one you probably never thought you'd be interested in, but when you have your own child, that all changes. When babies are newborn, they don't poop like everyone else. In the womb, they were learning how to drink by swallowing the amniotic fluid around them, so their little system has been saving up this special kind of poop for when they are born. It's called *meconium*. Honestly, it is the stickiest dark-colored stuff you can imagine! Luckily, you'll get some good instruction in the hospital on how to hold the baby's legs out of the way while you're wiping. Although I am a mother of girls, I learned a good tip of popping a cloth over a baby boy's "willy" so he does not wee on you while you are changing him. All babies seem to love the feel of air on their butts, and they often decide to poo or wee again just when you've put a clean diaper under them on the change table. It's like they know this will annoy you and they do it as a joke.

Once the meconium is all out of their systems on the third up to the fifth day, baby poop turns yellow. Then it's not so bad and definitely not as stinky. This is from the milk they're drinking, and it's going to stay like this until they start eating solid foods. Then things change and it all becomes like normal poop, and starts to smell too. That may sound disgusting, but this is your child. By the time that happens, you will be an expert diaper changer, so it will not bother you.

At the hospital, they used to tell me that you have to change the baby every two hours. So I followed their advice to the letter, but then I felt like I was throwing away clean diapers, so I started changing the baby every two to four hours, depending on how full the nappy was. It's one of those things you learn as you go. The important thing is to change them after they've pooped as quickly as possible so they don't develop diaper rash.

The Diaper Revolution

At the hospital, nurses teach you lots of practical things about how to care for your baby. Things like how to change nappies, bathe your baby, and dress it. Your baby seems so fragile, and learning how do all this on a real, live person isn't as simple as you think. Watching the videos when I was off with my broken leg definitely helped, but there's a big difference between your own tiny newborn and the baby in the video. In a few weeks' time, you'll be a pro. But those first few times are terrifying!

These days my friends and I take diapers for granted. Once you've got the knack and you're no longer scared of moving your baby around, they're very easy to use and, my goodness, they make life easier. Wrap up the little stinky parcel and throw it in the trash. Goodbye forever! Take the baby with you wherever you want to go and sort messes out in the bathroom. It's so easy. Of course, society is only just beginning to learn that disposable may not be so great, and our children may be angry with us about our throwaway lifestyle when our trash really starts to affect the planet's life cycles.

Things weren't always so convenient for women with infants and toddlers. For example, back when my mother first had children, nappies were nonexistent. They were such a revolution that Mom actually remembers the year they arrived: 1973. But of course, that didn't mean they were widely available. Instead, what women in this part of the world used to do was swaddle the newborn baby's chest and arms using one cloth and swaddle the legs using another cloth, while leaving the butt of the child exposed. The child's crib would then have a sandpit inside of it, just like a cat's sandbox. Every time the child soiled the sand, it would be changed. This is really hygienic and eco-friendly, but it didn't make it easy to travel with the baby. Back in those days, however, a woman's life was mostly at home, so that was less of an issue when the baby was small. When moms did need to go out and about with the children, or when the infants grew older and more mobile, they had to come up with their own solutions.

To make her own solution, my mother would buy cotton fabric from the "*lailam,*" a merchant who used to pass by in the neighborhood. Those kinds of merchants were more common in those days, because women couldn't always leave the house. My father was away on military service for long periods of time, so my mother had no one to take her to the souk. Her neighbors were kind and would help bring in almost everything she needed, while the lailam knocking on the door meant she could buy some of the other things she wanted to see before she bought. The lailam sold fabrics, perfumes, children's clothing, and other women's products. My mother would choose the fabrics, sew their edges, and use them as diapers. She remembers when she found nylon-lined underwear in pink and blue, which she could use as wraps for the padding. She would then wash the padding when dirtied. But one happy day, the neighbors bought her some disposables, and she never went back to the cotton wraps again.

The lailam is a fading tradition. With our malls and precincts and more personal freedom for women, we don't need door-to-door salesmen any longer. They really reflect a different time in our past that some people might feel nostalgic for. The lailam filled a real need in society and, in some ways, it is sad to see such traditions relegated to the pages of a history book. In a way, I think online shopping became our modern day lailam.

I Have No Idea What Time It Is

The first few days and weeks with a newborn are a rollercoaster. When your baby first comes home, she doesn't know the difference between day and night. She doesn't know what mealtimes are or even how to hold up her own head. Your baby can only focus about 30 centimeters away and will sometimes, very cutely, go cross-eyed as she learns how to focus at different distances. And the only way your baby has to tell you that something is wrong is by crying.

The problem is that you don't know which reason she is crying for at first. Is she hungry? Does she need a change? Is she lonely? Did she hear a noise that scared her? After a while you might stop knowing whether it's day or night yourself. If you're doing this by yourself and especially if you are breastfeeding, you will learn how to sleep in short bursts and to have your own checklist of needs to run through when she does cry. Is there a bad smell? Change her diaper. Have a cuddle? Is she rooting for milk? There you go.

I, for one, was losing my mind with my first child. I was so desperate to understand her in the beginning that I bought a device that encoded her cries and would tell me why she was crying. I do not know how accurate this device was, but I felt better thinking I knew the reason for the cries, as I was going insane. The device takes around twenty seconds to "encrypt" the cries. I remember Saeed was in the room once, Shereena was screaming, and I was just looking at the device waiting for it to give me an answer. Saeed was baffled by the idea that I would let the child scream until a battery-operated device told me why she was crying. But sometimes as a parent, you actually buy useless stuff like that just to get some reassurance!

Most parenting in the early weeks consists of watching your baby lie there, panicking when she cries and frantically going through your checklist until she stops! Most experts agree that babies are too small to follow a routine until they are around twelve weeks old, so the best advice is to relax, follow their lead, don't plan any big events, and learn how to be a family together with your child. You may not know whether it's night or day sometimes, but you will get there, even if it feels very tough for a while.

It's hard to learn to mother well, and it's even harder when you're exhausted. You are recovering from birth, either vaginally or through a C-section. Either way, you need rest. It all depends on your lifestyle, but I would suggest getting a night nanny if you don't have anyone else to help out. Give yourself the time you need to recover, knowing that other people are there to stay on top of the cleaning and nighttime feeds or changes. Yes, this can be expensive. But you are worth it! On "Friends," Rachel's mother told her, "You can't do this alone!" The woman was right.

Baby Business School

In every movie or TV show with an expecting couple, there has to be a scene at a Lamaze class. Phil and Vivian Banks went to one on an episode of "Fresh Prince of Bel-Air" and Ross, Carol, and Susan went to one on an episode of "Friends," among many others. The goal of a Lamaze class is to educate women about the basics of pregnancy and childbirth, as well as to give them strategies to cope with the newborn baby. In the West, fathers attend these classes to ensure their partner that when she is in doubt, they will be there to support her and that they are in this together. Fathers are also taught the correct breathing techniques to practice with their partner during labor.

As the United Arab Emirates is becoming more diverse year after year, classes such as Lamaze, prenatal yoga, and even prenatal emotional support groups are becoming popular. Those classes are open to everyone, of course. They are not mainly targeting Emiratis. The problem for me and many of my friends back in 2014 when I was expecting my first was that fathers were usually encouraged to attend these classes, which could be uncomfortable for women who wear abaya and shaila. Although I wished that such classes were available for abaya-clad women alone, I thought it was nice for fathers to take part in the process of bringing a new life to the world! And because attending these classes felt somewhat awkward for me back then, I learned everything I needed to know from books, DVDs, and YouTube instead.

After the baby is born, another modern option that is now available in the UAE is mother and baby classes. There are also good bonding activities that you can try with your infant, such as baby yoga or baby swimming. There are even cute classes with music and games. I was lucky to live close to a place that offered such classes for children as small as six weeks old. The classes they offered for babies were designed around their visual, audible, and spatial needs and strengthen both their minds and souls. My two older girls enjoyed attended those. However, the coronavirus pandemic forced the place to shut down, depriving my youngest, Alia, or enjoying these interactive baby classes. So get on the Internet, search for the nearest class, and have fun with your baby!

Who's the Mom Around Here?

I was so tired and so emotional in those early weeks. I had prepared so much for my first child's arrival when I was pregnant, so I knew what I was supposed to do and I just wanted to apply everything that I had learned and start being a mother to my child right away. But I felt like everything the people around me were telling me contradicted what I read. It made me so confused. Why would they be saying something different from the books? Who was right and who was wrong? I knew I trusted the authors. I trusted their expertise and experience and the scientific studies they based their tips on, and I just wanted to apply what I had learned from them.

Advice for moms-to-be and new moms comes to us from every direction: from previous generations in the family and friends remembering what they did and what they'd been taught by the generations before them, or from books telling us about the way other parents around the world approach parenting, or from scientifically measured and assessed data, doctors, psychologists, sociologists, and researchers who have observed pregnancy and parenting and have analyzed the data to produce their conclusions. In books, the authors justify and explain the reasons for what they advise—it's never just "because that's how it's always been." I read somewhere that in medieval Europe, they used to think that disease was caused by bad smells, and people carried posies of flowers to sniff in order to stop themselves from getting sick. Just because something has always been done one way, doesn't make it right. If doctors hadn't discovered bacteria, life today would be very different. And not in a good way. And speaking of bacteria, being a mother makes you wonder about so many things that could be remotely related to being responsible for a human life. That is why one day I found myself reading a book that talked about how penicillin was discovered. That book may have been dull, but I just had to know!

When I had Shereena, I found myself being confronted by people I love giving me advice that totally contradicted what I had learned from the books and that left me not only very upset but also confused. The pressure of having a newborn soul to look after is huge enough! A new mom does not need that added pressure of being made to feel that she is incapable or is doing a horrible job.

One perfect example of how the advice I got from different sources varied was about what to do immediately after the baby is born. Today, most of the books recommend skin-to-skin contact as much as possible from as soon as the baby is born. But many family members and friends were telling me no, don't do that, don't teach the baby to be in your hands all the time. You have to leave the baby in the bassinet, do not carry it, and so on. They said, "Don't teach her that every time she cries, you'll pick her up." This is the polar opposite of what I read in the books!

The experts in the books say that babies need us to hold them close and comfort them. It's the first time for the baby to be outside in the world. The baby is scared, and that's why she cries. They recommend that the baby be picked up whenever he or she cries to feel safe. That's one of the things I got angry about. It felt right to comfort my new baby, and I disagreed with relatives right there in the hospital. I remember showing how irritated I felt from the ongoing advice, which caused a few of my visitors to leave early and my mother to pack her stuff and leave the hospital when she had planned to stay with me until the baby and I were discharged. That was hard. I respect my mother, but you have to do what feels right for your child. I was now the mom in this situation, so I had to trust my instincts. My mom was upset, but that's only because she didn't understand the rationale behind what I had read.

For my second delivery when I had Mahra, I booked a very big room at the hospital that had a guest room inside. It was lovely, as it was like a hotel suite. Mom did stay with me that time and helped out. This time around, I think she recognized that I knew what I was doing, and I decided that she just wanted to be part of things. I also learned to nod and smile when visitors walked in with an excessive amount of advice.

In my culture, the newborn baby's grandmother helps out a lot. The grandmother usually looks after the new mother and the new baby at the same time, giving both of them the attention and help they need. But I did not have that when I had my firstborn, Shereena. I chose to stay in Abu Dhabi—as I mentioned, my husband was going to National Service just three weeks after my delivery. Therefore, it was just the two of us for twenty days with a newborn baby. At that time, I did not have a nanny or even a housecleaner at home. I was doing the cleaning and the washing by myself, which included the baby's bottles and clothes, until Saeed left and I moved in with my parents for three weeks. During these three weeks, Saeed was not allowed to contact us, and I was worried sick. What made it hard for me was knowing that he was worried sick about us, too. I really felt alone when he left, and that affected me a lot. I wish I had organized more help before the delivery, but who knew things would end up being so hard to manage! One of the reasons I wanted to write this book was to help other women like me understand that there is no shame in getting outside help when you have a new baby. If you need a night nurse or a nanny, get one. If you decide you can't manage the housework, get a cleaner or a maid. You are recovering from the major physical trauma of childbirth, and you will need to rest so you can be the best mom you can be.

Will You Ever Have a Normal Life Again?

For the first week or so, your baby will sleep a lot and most of it will happen during the day. You will discover that your baby "wakes up" a bit after the first week or so. It's as though she's realized she's not in the womb anymore and wants to be awake all the time! Now is a good time to try to learn a routine with your baby. Lots of books suggest that you should "teach" your baby a routine. I think it's more of working one out together, a routine that is right for both of you! And remember, the routine you develop is only going to work for a while. As babies grow, they don't need to eat as often, so that changes the routine. Plus their naps get longer, which changes the routine, and they might start having fewer naps, which changes the routine again. The best bit is that they sleep more at night, but not every baby is good at that. I have a friend whose child did not sleep through the night until she was four years old! Don't worry, though—that is very rare. It is certainly possible to get your baby to sleep for periods of four or five hours at a time after a few months. Then you will be able to get some longer sleep yourself and start to feel human again.

    I was desperate to get my daughter to stay in bed longer, which is why I did a bunch of ridiculous stuff that I'd read about on the Internet. One thing I read was to use anything that had lavender in it, from Dettol, to room sprays, to diffusers, to pillow sprays, to lotions, to bath bombs. I used it all until, at some point, my husband thought the house smelled like "hashish," which got me wondering where he might have smelled that! Once he took his pillow and slept in the living room because it was the only place that was not drenched in a lavender aroma. I admit that I overdid it, and no, it did not keep her asleep longer!

In my situation, I had the added fun of having a husband who doesn't sleep like other people. He sleeps whenever he feels tired, whether that is 5pm or 5am. His whole family works that way, so it made it tricky to encourage Shereena into a more standard routine. In the end, I gave in and did the same. Whenever he said he was going to bed, we all did. But I tried to keep a bedtime routine around 6pm with a bath, a bottle of milk, and bedtime story unless we had all gone to sleep earlier! When our second and third daughters came along, they just had to join in.

The only problem for me was that sometimes I really needed to stay up late due to social events even though my babies persisted in waking up really early and going to sleep really early, too. At some point, you might need to accept that your old habits and life of going out have to change while your children are small. Small children are naturally early risers. They wake and sleep with the sun. I have noticed that other people who've had children aren't at social events much anymore, either. I guess we don't notice what is absent until it affects us!

One of the strangest pieces of advice I got was that the baby doesn't need a bath every day. Here, my mother disagreed. She said that the baby needs to bathe every morning so she will be able to take a good afternoon nap, and it was totally true. There is no magic formula for a baby routine. The best thing to do is to match your routine to her preferred time to wake up or go to sleep, then after a few months, you'll find a routine that works for your family.

I would say, read everything you can about routines and have some ideas about what to expect when your baby reaches certain milestones. You can use this to plan your routine. But be prepared to forget it all, or at least adapt it, if it doesn't work for your situation; otherwise "the routine" will just become another burden.

Too Much to Do

One of the big tricks as a new parent is working out how to fit everything in. Your diary becomes full just with ensuring the family are all fed, clothed, washed, and where they should be! Remember that children need their mothers to be healthy and happy. They can sense if things are wrong. So ensure you include time for exercise, to visit the hairdresser, go to the mall, see your friends, and relax.

My mother told me that I needed to make a schedule for the baby right from day one, and this matched the advice in lots of the books. I was advised to think about her sleeping time, the timing of her feeds, when she was going to be bathed, and so on, and everything had to fit around her schedule. I followed the schedule and everything was fine. This is where using a nanny made a world of difference. To keep my lifestyle the way I needed it to be, having a nanny and someone to help manage the house was essential.

My best advice is to aim for a routine, but keep it flexible. Planning and being organized are how to keep sane, but don't let your plan become a rod to beat yourself with. If it stops working, find a new one. Eventually, your children will start nursery or school and things will settle down.

Getting a Good Night's Sleep

After reading lots of different books with lots of different theories about how to look after a baby at nighttime, Saeed and I prepared our first baby's crib in our room. Babies do not know about night and day. When they wake up in the dark, they are often scared. They are also probably hungry or they need a clean diaper. The easiest way to help yourself have the most sleep for all of you is to have the baby in the same room for a while. Set up a diaper-changing station right near the crib and have a comfortable chair to feed her in with low light.

To help your baby learn the difference between night and day, you need to use routine to help you. Make sure your behavior is different when the baby wakes in the day or in the night. During the day, when the baby sleeps it should be in the living area and there should be some noise happening. You should greet your child brightly and take her somewhere to feed, change, and then play. This will help the baby learn that daytime is bright and noisy, but she can sleep safely through that. The opposite should happen at night. The room should be dark, with only dim lights. You should talk in a quiet voice or not at all. Try not to chat to your baby at night, as this will be too stimulating for them. Quiet cuddles, soothing hugs, and rocking them are good to reassure them, but put them back in the crib once you have fed them. Only change a nighttime diaper if it is wet through or you can smell it needs to be changed. Feeling the air on their legs and bottom will wake them up more, which you don't want.

By having Shereena in our room, we managed to avoid the horrors of complete sleeplessness that I had heard about from other people. Many people told me that I would not be able to sleep at all when the baby arrived. It scared me, so I was glad it turned out not to be true! We grew to love her being there. It is reassuring to hear your baby sleeping when you go to bed yourself, and you enjoy having her near you. Shereena had her own room when she was almost a year old, and Mahra joined her sister at the age of two months.

Bath Time

When a baby is born, it often has some white sticky substance on it, and it has a clip over the stub of the umbilical cord. For the first twenty-four hours or longer, it is normal not to wash the baby but to keep it in clean swaddling. When you and your baby are ready, the nurses at the hospital will show you how to wash the baby safely. There are special bath seats to put in a sink or bath so that the baby won't slip under the water by accident. For my first daughter, I had a bathtub that I put on the floor in the middle of the room. I usually put a towel under it to avoid getting the floor wet and slippery. For Mahra and Alia, though, I bought a standing bathtub called a "bathinette," which looks almost like a changing table. I found it easier to use and it saved me the back pain. You fill the tub with warm water and wash the baby without leaning over, then there is a little pipe to drain the water away. Some even have lids that double as changing tables. This can be a good idea, especially if your back hurts after the pregnancy and birth.

There are lots of choices and controversy about the best products to use. Babies are so delicate, and we want to avoid putting chemicals on their skin. Look for organic products, or ones with minimal amounts of chemicals. With any product (or new food), make sure you test a small bit first, in case your child has a reaction to it.

To be completely honest, I was so obsessed with baby skincare products that I tried almost every brand out there, some shipped in from overseas and some purchased from the local grocery store. It took me a while to stop being lured by new brands and settle with the most convenient, mild, and gentle products that I could put my hands on within a few minutes' drive.

How to Mom in Public

I took my first child, Shereena, out when she was four days old. That day, I had an appointment at the hospital with a lactation professional to try to teach me how to breastfeed (I was still insisting, even though I was told I have flat nipples). After doing my best at the appointment without success, I got into the car with my husband and was again upset that I could not do what seemed to be the simplest, most basic job in motherhood. Because I was upset during the car ride and not focusing on the road, I suddenly realized that my husband was pulling over next to ZUMA—he was taking me to lunch at one of my favorite restaurants to cheer me up, with a four-day-old infant. Luckily, she slept the entire time and I did not have to "mom" for one second.

I remember wanting to go out to breakfast with my sisters one morning. I thought I'd just feed three-week-old Shereena and put her in the stroller, so she'd sleep the entire time and I'd chill with my sisters. However, as soon as we reached the restaurant, my daughter started crying. When I lifted her up from the stroller, she proceeded to vomit all over me. Definitely not the chilled-out morning I had hoped for!

I also remember going out with one of my closest friends, Asma, one day and we were going from one changing room to another because my baby wouldn't stop crying. The mall had, I think, six changing rooms and we visited each one of them so I could try to feed and comfort her. But she would not settle at all. I had so many images of myself enjoying shopping trips with my daughter in the stroller, but it was much harder than I had imagined.

Being a mom in public turns out to be really hard work. You feel like everyone is judging you and staring at you if your child makes some noise. It makes some moms give up trying to go out. But it is important to find a way to go out or you can become very isolated. The trick is to learn when your child wants to nap and to eat and time your trips around that as much as you can. The problem is that most babies like to sleep in the car, so instead of sleeping while you look around the shops, they wake up and want to play. It is a lot easier when your baby is older and you can switch the baby's position so she can look around. Newborns have to lie flat until their necks and backs are strong enough to sit up for a while. When they can do it, the baby can be quite entertained by looking at the things in the shops, too. The only problem is when they start to grab things!

The Perfect Mom

Society has a lot of expectations around what a good mother is and isn't. There are expectations from our families and the traditional Gulf culture, as well as from the international culture we find in our cities these days. There is a massive problem that many of these expectations contradict one another: "Good" mothers stay at home to care for their children, but "good" mothers also have full-time jobs. "Good" mothers have children, who know how to behave perfectly in every situation, and they do not shout at their children in public; they are quiet and demure. It is all so unrealistic. Honestly, if I think about all the ways I'm supposed to be a good mother, I would need to be some kind of saint with multiple personality disorder to make it work.

Having More Than One

Are you the kind of person who has always imagined having a large family? Or did you never think you'd become a mother at all? Or maybe, like me, you are somewhere in between. I always imagined I would have four or five children who would grow up together and have a strong sibling bond. After having my third child, I decided that six is the perfect number.

To have a good balance between being pregnant, nursing, and caring for an infant and then the next child, we planned a two-year gap between them. And the age difference between my first two daughters, Shereena and Mahra, is two years and four months, while the difference between Mahra and Alia is three years and three months. The good thing is that I can see that my daughters growing to be very close, they're very friendly with each other, and they play with each other all the time. I feel like if there were a big age difference, they wouldn't be as close.

Also, if you have children very close in age, you may not be able to go out with friends socially or continue your job. Some women are okay with that. They want to work only until they find the right man to settle down with. But you may find that when the children go to school, you become bored. Having a small business can be one option for women in this situation, and there are many opportunities to pursue careers these days. And with good childcare in the preschool years, it is perfectly possible to have a family and a nice work-life balance.

When your second child comes along, you may be very surprised to find that he or she doesn't react the same way as your first baby. The routine you worked out with your first baby might not suit this little person. Babies have a distinct personality from the moment they are born. Some need to be cuddled all the time. Others are more independent. Do not expect them to want the same routine, to like the same food, or to enjoy the same activities as their elder siblings.

A second child changes the family dynamic. When you have just one child, you might feel guilty for making them wait a moment for you to finish your task before you pick them up when they cry. Or you might feel guilty for staying late to finish a project at work and missing their bedtime. When you have two or even more, your feelings of maternal guilt reach a whole new level. The sad thing is that with Shereena, up until I had Mahra, when I would go out with her alone, we would play together and she would have my full attention. I was always the mom in the playpen with her kid, even when I was pregnant. Because it is almost impossible for me to go out without having both of them with me, I feel I have deprived Mahra of this kind of quality time with just the two of us.

Spending time just one-on-one with each of your children is hard to manage, but it is important. Once Mahra was sick, and I had to pick her up from nursery during the day. The next day she didn't go in and I didn't go to the office, either. I stayed with her and I worked from home. But I decided to take her out to breakfast with me so she wouldn't be stuck at home all day long. She was very cute and very calm, sitting down in her stroller eating what I gave her, not crying at all, just looking at people. I felt guilty that I had not had this experience with her before, while I used to have it a lot with Shereena. It was a big realization for me. Having more than one has deprived me of giving one child my full attention.

It can be easy with multiple children to let yourself just pay attention to the dominant ones. Shereena will always be the type of person who would pull my face towards her to make sure I listen to what she's saying. Or she'd say, "Mommy, look at me!" She loves being the center of attention, whereas Mahra is more placid and can get overlooked. This makes me feel really bad, but it is something I consciously try to push back against. It does help to know

I'm not the only one with this issue. A friend of mine told me about her experience with her two children. She said, "Our two-year-old was instantly jealous of his little sister. It was dreadful after she arrived. I would be feeding the baby and sometimes he would stand and wee up and down on the carpet in defiance. He knew I couldn't get up and stop him. It was his way of rebelling, and of making sure I was watching him and not having a loving moment with my daughter."

The most practical difficulty when you have more than one child is getting out of the house. With one, it is still relatively easy to go out. With two, and especially with a toddler and a preschooler, you need either a double stroller or two adults to go anywhere. Basically, you need another pair of hands. Having two kids at home completely stopped me from going out with my children all by myself. I'd rather have my husband or the nanny with me, because I found it very stressful to go out with both of them until Mahra reached the age of two. I always imagined Mahra crying while Shereena was having a tantrum and me standing right there not knowing what to do. I didn't want to put myself in that situation. The idea of it filled me with dread.

If you are pregnant with your second child, one great thing to do is to get some research done now. I know I come off like a nerd in this book, but I am obsessed with books. You get so much more from them than from just reading online. I like to highlight useful sections and tag the pages so I can find things easily. It can feel good to flick through the pages of a few books in the evening after your child has gone to sleep and you have a few quiet minutes.

But you should also seek out books for your child. This is the best trick: you want books about being a big sister, or having a brother or a sister, or having a sibling. I think there were like five or six that spoke about the same topic but in different scenarios, and I would read them to Shereena every night until she accepted the idea that a baby was coming and she was going to be a big sister and going to help me. I read the same books to both my daughters while pregnant with my third, which prepared Mahra to what was coming. That's why

I think there isn't jealousy between them. Shereena still loves attention, but I wouldn't call it jealousy. She loves her sisters very much, and so does Mahra. I feel like these books really make a difference.

If you want an opinion about how to space your children. I think the right time to have a second child is two to three years after the first one. At least have the first two close together, so they form a close relationship as they grow. And then you can have a break of a few years and then have another two who would be friends and so on. That's how I see it.

My own experience was quite different growing up. Because I wasn't part of the plan, the age difference between me and my nearest sibling is six years. But happily, we were very close. Even now, this brother, Rashed, is one of the closest siblings to me. Maybe a bigger age gap worked because I was the baby of the family, or it might have been because he had Mom to himself while he was in pre-school age and didn't feel his position was under threat from the new baby. Mom was able to focus on the baby without feeling like she was neglecting an older child. But I still feel the right time to grow your family is when the first child is two to three years old because they are more likely to enjoy playing together as they grow up.

Routines with More Than One

If you space your children two years apart, there is one issue that you might regret. Children tend to be ready to toilet-train around two years old. Some people say it can be done earlier and try to force it. The problem is that the child has to want to do it or it just won't work. You can no more force a child to learn to use the toilet than you can force her to learn to speak before she's ready. With infants each step is at the right time for them. So you may find that you are bringing home a newborn at the same time that you are toilet-training your first child. That is a tough combination. But if you have the right help in place, it should not affect you too badly.

On a day-to-day basis, the routine tends to fit around the older child's needs. Maybe this is why second children tend to be more easygoing. For us, bath time used to be before bedtime when Mahra was tiny, I mean right before bedtime, and I still follow that routine now with baby Alia. Lots of people do this and the bath becomes a signal for the baby that they will be going to sleep for the night soon.

So their schedule would be, for all three of my children coming back from nursery and school, playing for a while, then bathing, then having dinner, reading a bedtime story and then going to sleep. But I found it difficult because they get really tired from nursery, from playing and so on. This would make them really fussy earlier than bedtime. So sometimes I would bathe them in the morning to save myself the end-of-day agony. My children love playing in the water together. I think it's really cute!

In our home, Shereena and Mahra sleep in one room together, and they sleep next to each other in adjacent beds ever since Mahra was two months old. When Mahra was younger, she used to wake up, stand on the end of the bed screaming, so Shereena also wakes up. That was a daily occurrence; before crying and calling for me, she used to scream and yell for Shereena to get up. Then she would laugh that she woke her sister up. This happened every single day until she turned three years old and learned to walk to the living-room and switch on Netflix all by herself whenever she opens her eyes. I feel that as long as we all get a good number of hours of sleep, it is okay. I used to be extremely particular about how things were going to be when I became a mom. But I have come to realize that there are many things that are out of my control. Once I knew I could not control my children's every action, it became much easier to forgive their behavior or to relax when something didn't work out exactly as I'd planned. They are little people, not robots or tamable animals!

Eventually, I found a routine that seemed to work for everyone. In the morning I dropped my kids off, I went to work nine to five and then spent time with them until they went to bed. In the evenings and after bedtime, I tend to take care of personal errands, if any, or just curl up with Netflix or a book until I dozed off myself. I started scheduling salon appointments and social meetups during the weekend, when the children would be on playdates.

To make our routine work, Saeed and I make sure someone is there to watch the children, and we have to plan things in advance a lot. Or at least I do plan things in advance, as my husband is not a planner at all!

Since Shereena started going to "big girls' school," as she calls it, we have realized we need to change the routine. Saeed, as a modern Emirati man, will fetch Mahra at the end of the day from nursery and be home by the time Shereena's bus gets there at 3:30pm. I take care of the morning drop-offs, and then work until 5pm. Then I will head home and spend time with them until they sleep. If we weren't very good at coping with change, life as a parent would've been much harder. Children change so much as they grow up—even monthly or weekly at the beginning, and the routine has to change with them. It is impossible to plan things too much, as the baby may have completely different needs every day.

Getting the Right Help

Since I did not move in with my parents right after being discharged from the hospital when I had my first child like most Emirati moms do, I was under a lot of pressure to do everything myself. At first I really wanted to do it all. I felt like this was the right thing. I had planned how I wanted everything to be and I did a lot of research, so I felt confident with coping and looking after my child.

What I had not considered was that here in the UAE we have a specific lifestyle that demands a lot of help, especially as working moms. I think we are expected to look flawless all the time, with perfect makeup and perfect outfits from the minute you give birth. It is a lot of pressure, so when you add caring for an infant to the equation, it can easily feel like too much weight on your shoulders.

The reason why I believed I could do everything by myself—washing, cleaning, taking care of the baby, and looking flawless—is because I was influenced by TV and the Internet showing the mom who does push-ups with her child on her back, or one who gets the beach body a few weeks after giving birth. I was so convinced that I could do that too that I did not want to admit that it was hard when people told me "you can't." I wanted to prove everyone wrong, not thinking objectively of how our lifestyle, the weather, and the people might put that goal out of reach. Yes, my mother and my grandmother did it—but they did not have a full-time job or the options available to us now.

Only a few days after bringing Shereena home, I realized that our lifestyle's demands make the Western style of parenting I saw in the media unfeasible. I don't mean the well-groomed mommy with a cropped top flaunting her six packs while pushing a three-month-old baby in his stroller, because that's unrealistic for every culture out there. I am talking about the new exhausted mommy look. You know that look of a new, drained mother sometimes projected on television? Think about Miranda from *Sex and the City* right after she gave birth to Brady: messy, greasy hair, large sweater with stretchy pants, and a large bra with a front zipper, probably walking around with a vomit stain on her shirt. I thought this was only normal, which it is, and that it was going to happen to me, too. However, our lifestyle, not just here in the UAE, but in the GCC as a whole is different. We are expected to look clean and well-groomed because most new mommies around us are. We now have Arab influencers that, even though you might not be following them, pop up on your social media feed somehow. Some of those influencers are also new mothers who look like they could be walking down the runaway right after being discharged from the hospital. People around you who have babies and still look good have hired help! When there is a good chance you will deal with baby blues, sleeplessness, entertaining guests, and so on, it is okay to have some help. Find a good housemaid and a nanny. If you are able to make this decision and choose the right people while you are still pregnant, then that is even better! You can spend time choosing and even training the help to keep the house the way you prefer it.

I was brought up in a house that always had at least two house cleaners. I am not used to seeing piled-up dishes or laundry baskets. That is why whenever something is dirty, I wash it immediately. This was incredibly hard to manage once there was a baby in the house.

I decided to get help when Saeed was about to leave to the army. That is when I put myself first and thought: *I am tired. I am having baby blues. My husband is leaving to the army and will not be around for a long time. Why am I doing this to myself?* There is a verse in Quran that says: *"Allah does not burden a soul beyond that it can bear"* (Surat Al Baqara, Verse 286), which means that God does not lay a responsibility on anyone beyond his capacity. Yet I was doing it to myself.

Once I realized I needed help, I acted immediately and found a nurse through a local agency. This nurse cost a crazy amount of money. In fact, I spent almost all my salary to have her for three months, but I realized it was something I really needed. To be fair, it wasn't she who charged so much, it was the agency she came from.

The nurse started her duty right after Saeed went to national service and I moved in with my parents. She came each day from 10am to 10pm. This suited me very well, and my baby blues started to lift. She started to make me feel comfortable and gave me the freedom to enjoy this new stage of my life. I took long showers and used all the beauty products I had. I had time to go to the salon, catch up with friends over coffee, and just be human. I felt like I finally got the help I needed. I was rested and not stressed and was able to give my daughter the love and care she deserved.

Having the nurse gave me the freedom to take some time about choosing a nanny. The one I found was around fifty-four years old. She was very loving, very caring, and I could tell that she really loved my daughter. She stayed with us for around one and a half years. I would have kept her longer, except that I started to feel uncomfortable with her behavior. The following story is something you might want to consider when you're choosing a nanny.

Our first nanny was Filipino. This is very common here in the UAE. However, this particular nanny started to seem more like a grandmother to my child than an employee. This may have been because she was older. For example, she wouldn't follow my instructions or the doctor's instructions; she would do whatever they would do in her country. She thought she knew better. And that is unacceptable. I remember one time she came to me and advised me that when someone is sick and coughing, they should eat Vicks. Seriously. The vapor chest rub? Yeah, they would eat a spoonful of it! I was adamant that she should not do that with my daughter, but I know there were times when she did things I didn't agree with and I worried she would just feed my baby vapor rub anyway. That was when I knew I had to find someone else and let her go. You have to have complete faith in your nanny. After all, you are leaving your most precious possession with them.

My first thought when I chose that nanny had been that it would be good for Shereena to have a grandmother-type figure looking after her when I was at work. But after a while, she began acting like I was her daughter and she could tell me what to do with Shereena. The second nanny was also a mom, and she was very loving as well and caring. But this time, she was younger, in her thirties. She's still with us now, and we are very happy. This nanny follows instructions, and I know she follows exactly my style of parenting when I am not around.

I did not know how to treat the help until I went through six nannies / housemaids. Even though we have always had help at home, I was never the one in charge. When I hired my very first housemaid while still pregnant with Shereena, I decided to treat her differently from what people are accustomed to in this part of the world. Usually, housecleaners and nannies in the Middle East are not given the freedom they have elsewhere in the world. Back when I hired my first in 2014, some people still did not allow the housemaid or the nanny to own a mobile phone; she was to use the landline whenever she wanted to make phone calls (after taking her employer's permission). Also, days off are still frowned upon in some households. But when I hired someone, I decided to treat her with respect and like an adult. On her first day, I gave her my old iPhone, the WIFI password, and a day off every week. The topic of housemaids and nannies comes up at every gathering, and people feel the need to tell you what you should and should not do. I listened to others' beliefs. I checked her Facebook page every time she went out. I don't know why I felt the need to know where she was, but I did—until I discovered that she used to leave the house in the middle of the night wearing stolen clothes from my sister's closet. So maybe it was a good thing that I used to check? I don't know, I have mixed feeling about this, but I just had to fire her.

I kept hiring and firing until I realized that I should not listen to anyone's opinion on how I treat my help, and I decided to relax about the whole thing. There is somehow this notion that if you're in control of your help—if you don't let her go out, if you don't let her use your WIFI, if you don't give her any extra money on top of her salary—then you're just brilliant and know how to run a home. Well, I decided I don't want to be that version of "brilliant" and I don't want to be in control. I reached the ultimate peace of mind when I decided to just let go of all the extra pressure. As long as my house is clean, my clothes are tidy, my kids are being well taken care of, I don't care about anything else. With us, there is no such thing as a day off, because my help can stop working and go out whenever they feel like it. Just as we like to stay connected to our family and friends, it is their right to stay in touch while they are more than 5,000 miles away from their children. As long as they live with me, my house is their house, they can open the fridge and grab anything they want and ask for monetary support whenever they need it. Ever since I adopted this mentality, I have been happy with the people I have hired, I trust them, and they're also happy and they trust me. My children's nanny has been with us for almost three years now, she went on her biennial vacation for two months instead of one, and I even send her home whenever her children are sick. When I first hire someone, I give each a list of tasks that I needed them to do—some on daily basis, some weekly, and some monthly. This serves as a job description of what is expected of them. If everything is ticked off and done as required, they are free to go out, sleep, or do whatever they want, and this is exactly what I think everyone should do if they want peace of mind. Your help cannot read your mind. Write things down, explain to them, make up a schedule, and everything should go smoothly.

I am so happy that the government is doing its best to give hired help the rights they deserve. However, it will take a long time to change people's mentality to accept the fact that housemaids, drivers, and nannies should be treated the same way you'd want to be treated at work.

Back to Work or Not

Young Emirati moms tend to go back to work when their babies are around two to three months old. This is plenty of time to get to know your child and to get routines set up. But as a first-time parent, you have no idea how paranoid you can get. You worry about things you never considered before, so the idea of going to work and leaving your baby with a nanny fills you with dread. A popular solution has been to install security cameras. Moms sit at their desk with a channel tuned in on their phones, and if they can't see the baby they immediately fear the worst—or at least I did!

I had cameras set up at home and I felt a sense of enormous responsibility. It felt very stark and cold that I was leaving my child behind for a job. It felt like I was abandoning her. I had to make sure that she was alright the whole time. Somehow this translated into a need to be able to watch her. It seemed that if I could see her on the cameras, then somehow I was still actively parenting at that moment. I can tell you now it is almost impossible to get any work done if you try to parent remotely at the same time. It was awful. I became obsessed. I would sit at my desk at work with my cell phone permanently in front of me, or I would be in meetings presenting and the minute I would look at my phone and couldn't see my daughter, I would leave the meeting and call the nanny and ask her, "Why is the camera not working?" or "Why are you not in this room?" That is when I realized it had become obsessive and unhealthy. I am now extremely against installing these cameras at home except for security reasons on entrances, which I do not think we ever need to worry about considering that Abu Dhabi is the safest city in the world!

When I realized that I was starting to become affected and distracted at my job and that I wasn't achieving anything positive by simply watching Shereena all day, I knew I needed a different solution. That's why I decided to take her to nursery when she was one.

Find What Works for You

Most of the books I read were not aimed at women living in a desert climate. Their advice isn't suited to a country where, for most of the year, you can't sit outside in a park.. There was so much advice about going out with a baby. But here going out with a baby is very hard, because we can't just put a baby in a stroller and walk outside. It is often 50 degrees—the baby would get heatstroke. In the UAE, going out with a baby requires getting in the car, putting the stroller in, putting the baby in the car seat, and driving for a long time. If the baby starts crying, someone has to comfort them in the back seat. Then when you reach the place you are visiting, there is all the work of getting the stroller out of the car, setting it up, getting the baby in it, and so on. This is too difficult to do on your own, not impossible, but difficult.

For me, my ideal solution was to hire the nanny and to set up the right team of people around me so I could tend to the needs of my lifestyle and manage my new role as mom in a comfortable way. You may not want to think like this. I know I didn't before I had a child. I thought I'd be one of those moms who washes the bottles, does the laundry, takes care of the baby, and goes out with the baby while wearing perfect makeup and the nicest outfit around while also juggling a career. I had a very clear picture in my mind of what my life was going to look like. But reality can be quite a surprise, and I found my dream was unrealistic. I really felt that I needed to turn the situation around to create a good life for myself and my family. Once I came up with my home-help solution, I started to see how my life could be managed. Then my worries started to lift.

When I had my second daughter, I knew instantly that I would do the same again. A few months before giving birth, our current nanny came in so she could get used to my older daughter. I also had a housemaid at home to take care of all the cleaning and washing. So my baby blues were not as bad with my second daughter. I still felt them, I was still crying, but not as much as with my first daughter. And I felt more comfortable having people helping me with all the work.

There are a lot of practical considerations when you choose a nanny in the UAE, and one of the big factors for some parents is money. Getting nannies here in the UAE is very, very expensive. You have to pay the agency a fee on top of the salary of the nanny, and the amount you have to pay the nanny differs from one agency to another. It can really add up, so you need to be prepared for that. The agency fees include the cost of flying her from her country to here. Then you are responsible for her medical tests and her visa charges, her ID, and all of that. You are taking on an employee, so there are responsibilities that come with that as well. This person will be spending a lot of time with your child, so find someone you feel comfortable with and someone you respect and trust. And when you do, your life will seem smooth and stress-free.

Nurseries

I know this is controversial for a lot of Emirati families, but in my opinion the next step on from having a nanny is sending your child to nursery. When Shereena was one, I decided this would be better for her, even though my husband was against it.

For the first three months of her life, I was at home with Shereena on maternity leave. Then I went to work and she stayed at home with the nanny. Then when she turned one, I took her to the nursery. When I mentioned it to Saeed the first time, he was completely taken by surprise. No one in his family and nobody he knew had ever sent children that small to nursery or daycare. As he explained, he couldn't see the benefit of spending all that money when it is better for a child to be at home. We had the nanny already, and we had a camera so we could see what Shereena was doing during the day. Why did we need to change anything?

I explained my concerns about the granny-nanny who we had at the time and her changing attitude at home of trying to do things her way. I also explained how the camera was not a positive thing. What if, God forbid, the house was on fire? What if there was an emergency that the nanny was not capable of dealing with? Having the cameras installed at home also prevented me from working efficiently. I highlighted how research showed that children who attend nurseries start to perform better. Eventually, I convinced him it was the right thing for our family. Later on, and even now, actually, when he sees how she's social, how she's smart, and how she has this amazing vocabulary, he agrees that we made the right decision.

One of the benefits of enrolling a child in a daycare is exposing them to a lot of information, as opposed to the routine the child would have at home. For instance, when Shereena was only three years old, she used to talk about Neil Armstrong because she had a teacher who talked to the children as if they were grownups. She talked to them about space, about astronauts, about artists, and she opened up their minds and imaginations to interesting topics. I really love this nursery that I took her to, and I know my daughter would not be getting this kind of development at home with an iPad, a TV, and a nanny in the room being watched through a surveillance camera.

To help you know what to look for in a good nursery, I made a checklist:

1. First up would be **the safety of the facilities**. Is the facility designed with small children in mind? Have they baby-proofed, do they regularly disinfect the toys, are the children separated by age group, and are there enough staff for each age group? Children under one year old who can't walk need a ratio of one adult to two infants, while children who are four years old will be quite safe and well cared for with one adult around six children. Make sure you ask what the ratios are for different age groups and see if you are happy with their system.
2. Second would be **the cleanliness of the facilities**. When you walk in, how does it smell? If there is a whiff of vomit or poop, it is probably not a good place. I was shocked by the number of nurseries I visited where the smell made me gag and retch. Aside from being unpleasant, it suggested they were not sanitizing the surfaces well enough after accidents, and I would worry about what viruses my children would catch there.
3. The next most important thing is **the friendliness of the staff**. Small children need closeness, friendliness, and a loving relationship with adults to help their

development. Nursery staff should not have straight faces or an unwillingness to get down on the floor and play with the children. Watch the staff and how they interact with the infants in their care.

4. One more point to look at would be **the curriculum**. I enrolled Mahra, my second-born, when she was only three months old. At that age, I still expected her to have a curriculum that included activities to help her development: things like sensory play to help sensory development, exploration that helps motor skills development, tummy time, music, play, etc. I was very keen that the nursery where I enrolled my children did not simply feed the children and put them down for naps throughout the day!

There are some things that would make me instantly know a nursery was *not* the right place for my children:

1. I always asked about the staff turnover rate. I understand that it is important for children to interact with as many people as possible, but if the teachers change frequently, it is quite alarming. If a child gets attached to a teacher and that teacher leaves, then another teacher comes and leaves, I worry that the child might be heartbroken or start having separation anxiety. It is important to me that the staff stay for a long time. Staff who are well paid and well treated tend to stay in a job longer. They are also usually happier, and it is important that your children not be in a tense or unhappy environment.

2. I would ask the nursery to explain their disciplinary policy to me. Toddlers need to learn what behavior is acceptable and what behavior is not. But there are ways to teach this without yelling or humiliating anyone. If I noticed the staff yelling at children, my children would be out of there immediately! There are many long-term effects on children who encounter yelling or the wrong kind of discipline,

such as smacking. So check the nursery has a safe behavior policy that agrees with your own ideas about discipline. One of the reasons I decided to switch to a nursery while I was at work was that I read an article that showed children at nurseries have better behavior than those who grow up in other environments. Do your own research so you can make an informed decision.
3. A good nursery will develop a child's communication skills. This reduces frustration and improves behavior. Even if your little one can only say three to five words, if enrolled at a great nursery, your child will become a great communicator through gestures and facial expressions. Shereena's nursery prepared her for school. When she started school, everything seemed to be easy for her. She already knew all the alphabets, could count to twenty, knew all the colors, and knew basic math! She was also confident and did not cling to me at the morning drop-off. I saw other children screaming and kicking for their parents. I truly believe she would not have been so well-developed if she had been at home with just her little sister and a nanny every day while I was at work.
4. Another important area for me was the size of the nursery. You don't want to feel like your child will be lost in the crowd. Children need to make connections with the adults and have continuity. So the nursery can't be too big, but also it shouldn't be too small. It needs to have enough room to accommodate classes for different ages (three months to four years old), as well as the space to allow kids to play freely indoors and outdoors.
5. The childcare team need to make you feel comfortable with them. Talk to them and see if they're friendly. Are they committed to their jobs? Watch them tell the children a story so you can see how the children react to them. Storytelling skills are important for this age group. With all this, you should

be able to tell if they are passionate about what they do.
6. The final thing to consider when you are in the process of choosing the nursery is the location. Make sure it is either close to home or close to your office in case of an emergency.

Many things put me off the other nurseries. Some smelled horrible. Others had Arab teachers speaking in broken English to children, which really irritated me. I mean, if you can't speak English well, just don't speak to children in English at all.

So I went all around the nurseries near my office, all around the nurseries near my house, and I just loved the nursery that I chose. When I walked in, I knew this was the place I wanted my daughter to be, a place I could trust and feel comfortable leaving my daughter for the whole day.

What I do not understand is modern-day parents' obsession with cameras. If you say that your baby is at home, you will immediately be asked if you have installed cameras, and same thing happened when I chose a nursery. A lot of people were asking me, "Oh, do they have cameras? Can you see what she's doing the whole day?" No, they do not! And I'm happy that they don't! If they had them, I feel like I would start being this obsessive mother who keeps on looking at her child the whole time. That didn't work when they were at home, and it sure wouldn't work while they were at the nursery. I have to trust the people and the institutes I choose to take care of my children. If an incident happened, they would be able to show me the security-camera footage. I have never needed this, but it is reassuring to know it is an available option.

I chose a place that I'm comfortable with, and I was convinced they were going to take good care of my child. The minute I walked in, it felt like the right place. I think every mother should do that, whether it's a school or nursery or anything. I did the same thing when enrolling Shereena in a great international school in Abu Dhabi, the minute I walked in, I knew this was the place where I wanted her to be schooled. I could see that everyone was very disciplined, they have creative projects on display, and so on. I believe that gut feeling is really important when it comes to these things.

When we had our second daughter, Mahra, in fact even when I was still pregnant, I told my husband that this baby would be going to nursery right after my maternity leave. He could see how good it had been for Shereena, so Mahra went when she was three months old. A lot of people seemed a bit shocked. They asked things like, "What is she going to learn there?" and "Why are you taking her there?" A lot of people made jokes when they saw her on the way to or from nursery, like "Oh, she's going to college!" and other silly comments. I think this just shows their ignorance and is just another example of how society thinks it can judge mothers.

I know that even if I weren't working, even if I were at home and had nothing to do but look after those children, they would not learn as much as they learn at day care. In a social environment like that, they are exposed to a lot of people, a lot of faces, a lot of voices, a lot of languages. Even when Mahra was three months old, she had a French lesson and an Arabic lesson. Exposing kids to languages at an early age really helps them learn languages easily later.

One of the things I want to leave you with about nurseries in the UAE is just how much the children there learn to be sociable. My daughters have a wonderful level of confidence. They will go to anybody and smile and give hugs and converse. And I love that about them, and I appreciate how much of that comes from the hours they spent at nursery while I was at work.

Traveling with Your Babies

When your baby first comes home, it will be a mission to even leave the house to shop for food or go to the mall. There will be many days when you decide it is too hard and you simply won't go! There is so much to think about, from the diaper bag to the changes of clothes, the toys, the blankets, the stroller, the sunshade, and so on. Once you master that, then you might start thinking about going a little farther, maybe even on holiday.

The first overseas trip I ever took with a child was in 2015, when Shereena was nine months old. It was our second wedding anniversary and we wanted to go back to the Maldives, where we had gone on our honeymoon. The flight from Abu Dhabi to the Maldives is four and a half hours, which is daunting for a couple with a baby. So I purchased a few books about traveling with a baby so I'd be prepared.

I made sure to read every single word in each one of these books to ensure that I would have a smooth flight with a nine-month-old. I packed my carry-on, focusing on the things my child would need within the first hours of the trip: the two hours at the airport before taking off, the duration of the flight, and time travelling from the airport to the resort. So I thought, in my carry-on I would need:

- Three to four servings of formula and three to four clean bottles (my daughter had a bottle every three hours back then)
- Hot water to mix the formula
- A bottle of room temperature water also to mix the formula

- An extra outfit in case she threw up during that time or dirtied her clothes in any way
- Three to four nappies, as I used to change them every three hours on average
- Wipes
- Diaper cream
- A pack of tissues
- Some baby finger food for her to snack on
- One pureed meal to have at the airport before taking off

In the checked luggage, I packed what I thought she would need for the five days of the holiday. I never overpack. I always pack exactly what we need. That was fine for the travel, but when we arrived at the resort, I was stunned—not because of the beautiful views of the clear water and the amazing weather, but because the resort had prepared everything my daughter could possibly need. Knowing that we were arriving with a baby, they stocked our room with a crib with some soft toys in it, a range of baby products, and a bottle sterilizer! Yes, a bottle sterilizer! Their thoughtfulness really made this first trip more enjoyable and relaxing. I felt looked after and supported. For Shereena, it was her first experience on the beach. And she really loved it! We were able to relax as a family and enjoy the warm water and the views in comfort. I recommend finding a resort that is child-friendly, so you know you will have help while you are there.

On the date of the anniversary, Saeed and I went out for dinner. We arranged to leave our daughter asleep at the villa with a nanny, using the resort's babysitting service. We could enjoy our time together, knowing she was being watched over. The minute we were done with dessert, the restaurant got a call from the nanny saying, "The child is crying, I can't control her, please tell them to come back!" Of course, we went straightaway. Poor Shereena was really terrified because it was someone she had never seen before. A stranger was there instead of Mom and Dad! Next time, I would ask the nanny to come earlier so my child can meet her before going to sleep. That way, she might be less worried if she suddenly woke up while we're still out.

When I told people that I was traveling with my nine-month-old, they were generally negative and dismissive. The typical first comment was that traveling with a baby is such a hassle, and that I would have to pack a whole lot of things, such as a bottle sterilizer, which would take up half a suitcase. Other comments I received were like, "Poor thing, you will be dragging her through airports and she will be tired and will get sick." However, from my extensive research about baby products and baby-related topics, I read that we don't have to sterilize the bottles after every use! Sterilizing the bottle is meant to happen only when we first purchase it. Then washing the bottles with warm water and soap is sufficient. Ideally this should happen in a dishwasher, where the temperatures can be hot enough to do the job of sterilizing. But the people I know tend to sterilize the bottles after every use. I still do that out of peer pressure, but I am convinced that we don't have to sterilize them after every use! So during the time that we travel, I tend to be more lenient about this. If you want a travel-friendly method, try the one I found online and followed throughout all my trips with my children:

1. Fill the kettle provided by your hotel room and set water to boil. Meanwhile, wash out the sink, stopper, and faucet with hot soapy water, and rinse.
2. Once the kettle has boiled, rinse the sink, stopper, and faucet with boiling water. Refill the kettle and set to boil once more.
3. Fill up the sink with hot soapy water and wash the bottles, nipples, sippy cups, pacifiers, and any feeding utensils you want sterilized, then rinse with hot water.
4. When the kettle has boiled for the second time, pour the boiled water over washed items and swish around. Carefully remove items once the water has cooled and place on a clean towel to air dry.

Successful Trips

Because of the success of this first trip, we became more confident. When Shereena was fifteen months old, we took her to Kuwait, and that was a success, too, and a shorter flight. The good thing is that there is almost no time difference, so we didn't have to worry about jet lag. Next, we decided to brave a trip all the way to Europe (an eight-hour flight) and take a road trip across Ireland. Shereena was nearly two at this point, and I was three months pregnant with Mahra. Looking back, it is definitely easier to travel when the children are under one year old, because they need less entertainment and they are less mobile, so the flights are easier.

Ireland is a beautiful country, and Shereena was entertained because it looked so different from home. We went from Dublin to Belfast and Galway and visited beautiful old castles and enjoyed the rolling hills and mountains. Shereena had never seen cattle before, or so much green grass. She was fascinated by it all, which helped the car journeys. We spent two weeks traveling around, so there was a lot of time in the car. But we allowed Shereena to have an iPad, which helped the time pass when she became frustrated about being in the car seat. What made the trip work when I was exhausted from the pregnancy was that Saeed and I shared the childcare. Well, most of the childcare. If I was tired, my husband would always be there to help. He is the type of man who would wash the bottles, entertain the child, feed her, and do absolutely anything EXCEPT changing nappies. He would die before changing one!

Having two kids did not kill my wanderlust. I still wanted to travel and explore and see the world. The first trip I had with both children was to Kerala, in India. We arrived at

Cochin Airport after a four-hour flight, then had a two-hour drive to the resort. Mahra was only two months old, and Shereena was two years and eight months old. The resort was in a beautiful location on the lake. We spent almost the whole time in a villa with a pool. There are quite a lot of things you can do with small children in tow. We took a cruise across the lake the resort was on, we went fishing, and we spent many hours swimming with Shereena in our plunge pool. It was a very relaxing trip. In fact, Mahra spent most of it asleep. Of course, as she was only two months old, she had not had her full set of vaccinations, so it was important to ensure the resort was not in a high-risk area. India is beautiful, but it has its risks.

I was so keen not to overpack for this trip that I actually under-packed! I could see the level in the formula tub get lower and lower. I thought we were going to run out it, so I panicked! I tried to find a supplier that sold the formula she used, but I couldn't find anything close to where we were. Unlike the one in the Maldives, this resort was not helpful at all. But thankfully, the last serving of formula was given to Mahra on our flight back home and we managed not to starve our baby!

We took some beautiful trips when the kids were a bit older, as well. We traveled to Sri Lanka and celebrated Mahra's second birthday at a beautiful lodge in the middle of a jungle. The whole experience with jungle animals and staying at a tented lodge was very interesting to both of my girls, and we ended up having a blast. Another amazing trip we took was again to the Maldives that same year. You would think that such destinations were made for couples, but children do enjoy the water a lot, and a trip to such islands is the perfect getaway with children.

Road Trip Should Have Been a Nope Trip

By now, my confidence in traveling with infants was very high. But pride comes before a fall and we took a trip across Europe in 2017 that was quite different from the previous ones. I don't know what possessed us to book it. We took a road trip to Germany, Switzerland, Austria, Liechtenstein, France, and Italy. With two tiny children in the car. Shereena was almost three and Mahra was only five months old. What were we thinking?! If you have small children, I am sure you understand why this felt suicidal. During the hours and hours on the roads, Mahra cried a lot. We found some lullaby music that we played all the time in the car just to keep her quiet. I don't think I could bear to hear that tune ever again!

At one point when Mahra was crying a lot, I told my husband to stop the car and I got out with her for some fresh air. We just parked on the side of the road at a bus stop. I carried her over and sat there on the bench, trying to cheer her up and calm her down. Then, out of nowhere, next to my ear, I felt this heat and I heard a soft mooing noise. It was so close by, I freaked out! Where did this cow come from?! It was right behind me. Of course, I didn't want to make any sudden movement, just in case the cow decided to kick me or my baby. So I had to calmly walk back to the car like nothing was wrong. Looking back, it seems funny now. What is a cow going to do? But at the time, it was terrifying and I was very shaken.

We had picked possibly the worst age you could choose to travel with small children. Both of them were still in nappies, so they both needed to be changed across the day.

There were seemingly countless bottles and sippy cups to wash each day, plus they were both fairly mobile and alert. They needed to do more than sit still in a car seat for hours on end! They were bored so they cried, but we had to reach the next destination, the next hotel, so we couldn't just stop and let them out to play for long periods. It was totally draining, especially as I was on diaper duty. Endless, endless diaper changes in the back of the car. The process hurts your back and is so exhausting.

But that is not to say the trip was all bad. We did see some amazing sights and visit some fascinating, beautiful places. But when you travel with small children, you have to think about things you wouldn't have considered previously.

Looking back at pictures now, I long for those days. When you are in the middle of an experience of such kind, you start getting irritated by all the things that small children are either depriving you of or all the things they demand. However, when you look at pictures later on, you miss these moments.

Good Places to Visit with Kids

The following stories offer insights into the types of places that work, or don't work, for families with small children.

I remember walking up Sigmund-Thun-Klamm, a beautiful hiking path in Austria, while carrying Mahra. She was only five months old, so we couldn't put her down. I had her in my arms and I was worried about dropping her, so I was holding her really, really tight and close to my chest to the extent that when we went back to the car, my arms had gone numb. The path lets you see some amazing scenery, but it was not designed for people carrying children! It is narrow and some parts are uneven under your feet, so you have to be very careful. Shereena was with my husband, who had her up on his shoulders the entire time. It made me nervous. What if she slipped? But I trusted my husband to keep her safe. What made going through that hiking path even more difficult was that it was a rainy day, so the path was wet under our feet. I was really worried about falling and just tumbling down the mountainside. However, the views were really nice, and I am glad I got to experience that with my children and husband. It was a learning experience for Shereena, who saw things she had only read about in books, such as a waterfall, a river, mountains, and rocks. If you plan to go for hikes with your family or visit mountains with your children, I would recommend getting a sling for the infants and a safety harness for older ones, given how unsafe the steps were for little ones. You don't need to let it stop you, but planning will make it a better experience for you all.

Tegernsee, Germany, is a very nice place to visit with small children. There aren't many activities there, but being out in nature plays an important role in children's development. Shereena was greatly influenced by Peppa Pig at that time, so she would jump in a muddy puddle every time she saw one. It barely rains in our country, so for her rain and mud were a novelty, something she had only seen on the TV screen. It was fun and an adventure, not just wet and cold! Tegernsee was so green and our hotel was on top of a hill. The town had a big lake in the middle, which made the views breathtaking. Shereena was not so restricted as she usually is indoors. She had the freedom to run, scream, and have fun. It was liberating for her. Choosing a destination in a temperate climate with space for children to simply play safely outside is a great option for families from the Gulf.

One of my most memorable moments was our visit to the Lünersee in Austria. The minute we got out of the cable car and stepped out of the station, it took our breath away. It was extremely cold, so I had to use two swaddles around my baby. Shereena, on the other hand, wore my husband's sweater and he had to freeze! Such is the love for our children that we do things like this. Lünersee is by far the most beautiful scene I have ever come across in my life. The fact that there is such a huge lake that high up is mesmerizing. They had a little playground for children that included a slide and a swing, which Shereena enjoyed. I recommend taking advantage of cable cars to reach places with children. The countries in the Alps have plenty of them for skiers, but many of them operate in the summer months, too. This makes it pleasant for families to get to the tops of mountains and enjoy the great views.

In Italy, there are many mountain areas to choose from. Friends of ours recommend visiting the Lake Garda region in the Alps. You can use cable cars there, and the towns around the lake itself have many beautiful features. Malcesine Castle sits right on the lake and looks like it is from a fairytale. We didn't go there ourselves, but it seems to tick a lot of child-friendly boxes. On our trip, one of the few man-made places our toddler loved was Pisa. She was totally fascinated by the leaning tower. She couldn't decide whether or not it was going to fall on our heads at any moment. Even after we returned home, she went back to nursery and talked to her teacher about it. We explained that it was built on soft ground, which made it lean, and that is exactly what she kept telling everyone. I loved how she was fascinated by this and that she was able to learn from the things she did with us. That's what's beautiful about taking your children with you on trips. They explore, they see, they ask questions, and that definitely influences their development and how they see the world.

One place I didn't try to take the children was Abbey Library of St. Gall in Switzerland. I had studied this library and was eager to visit it. I'm the type of person who loves visiting museums and historical sites when I travel. To me, the most important things when visiting a new country are tasting the local food, learning about the culture, and picking up a few words of the language. I especially enjoy getting immersed in the local history through site visits. Unfortunately, that is very hard to do with children, as they get bored pretty easily. Children love visiting nature, as they can explore and touch things, but visiting historical sites is torture for them. They are not usually allowed to touch anything or run around; people want them to be quiet. So I knew I should leave them behind on this part of the trip. Luckily for me, the kids were asleep in the car as we pulled into the car park, so my husband offered to stay with them while I visited the library. Libraries are not really his scene, either, as he is not a fan of reading. So I went in by myself, and I was mesmerized. It felt like a special treat to have it to myself. We moms get so little time to ourselves! The library had Baroque architecture, something I had studied back in university, and my professor had talked to us specifically about St. Gall during my art history course. I am sure if the kids had been with me, they would have given me a hard time and I wouldn't have been able to take it all in.

How to Pick a Hotel

The most important thing for me when choosing a hotel was the size of the room. Since the four of us were in one room, it always had an extra bed for Shereena and a crib for Mahra. Knowing that hotels in Europe can be smaller than those in the Gulf or other parts of the world, I made sure to choose hotels that had large rooms, 45 square meters or bigger. That way, we would have plenty of space for the kids to move around, and comfortable space for all of us to rest.

It is also important for me to pick hotels that have a kids' club and a nanny service, in case we require help. I remember when we were staying at the Interalpen-Hotel Tyrol, we all got the chance to have fun. Shereena went to their massive kids' club that offered a lot of activities. We didn't have to stay with her, as they look after the kids themselves. At the same time, my husband went to the gym, and I was planning on hiring a nanny and visiting the spa. To my disappointment, I could not get an appointment. So the key learning here is to plan ahead for such times. I ended up putting Mahra down for a nap and enjoying afternoon tea and a book on the hotel room's terrace, which was delightful.

Planes, Trains, and Automobiles

Long journeys on planes are nobody's idea of fun. It can be a nightmare with small children. I always choose to fly at night, so we can encourage them to get some sleep. Ever since I moved to Abu Dhabi, I have been flying on Etihad. Since children under two do not have a seat of their own, I find it much easier to fly business class, as it is more spacious and comfortable, especially during long flights. The best place to sit is the first row, since it is the only place where you can assemble the airplane's bassinet, and it has more space for children to move (if they are allowed to). I was surprised to find out that Etihad actually have in-flight babysitters who will sit with the children and keep them busy with activities. It is an excellent service.

Always choose or hire a car that has lots of space. You need enough room to fit your cases, as well as two car seats. Ensure the hire company has reserved these for you, or take them on the flight if you prefer your own. If you could find a car with screens on the back of the front seats for the children to be able to watch videos, that would be excellent! All these small details will make any long journey more bearable.

One bit of good advice we got was about the stroller. We had been planning on taking the double stroller to fit both our girls. However, friends and family reminded me that the sidewalks in Europe are very narrow and wouldn't fit the double stroller. I had been to Europe before I became a mom, but I never paid attention to the sidewalks or people with strollers. Until you need to consider it yourself, you don't really think about these details. So we decided to get a compact stroller that fits in the airplane's cabin for our little one. Shereena walked most of the time. She only asked to be picked up a few times, so I think having only one stroller worked well for us.

Actually, a compact stroller is the best thing that has ever been invented for families on holiday. I cannot stress how important it is to have one with you when you travel. It really made my life easier. Mahra was asleep the entire time, and she was happy being pushed around the airport in the stroller up until we reached the airplane's seat. Thanks to innovative companies, double strollers are now available in compact size, which is perfect for families with two small children.

For Shereena, the airport itself was quite entertaining. She enjoyed standing by the windows looking at the airplanes. She was very quiet the entire time and the minute I felt like she was about to get fussy, I pulled out an activity from the busy bag I have prepared for her.

Keep Them Busy

I created a busy bag for Shereena to enjoy on trips. It contained coloring books, a notebook for her to scribble in, crayons, and two different puzzles that were suitable for her age. Shereena was not allowed to use an iPad until she was four years old, since I found she had come across some unsuitable videos on YouTube when I left her watching Peppa Pig one time at the age of two. I got her a portable DVD player instead, the one that looks like a laptop—super old school. Her favorite shows on DVD include universal favorites like Peppa Pig, Ben and Holly, and a Barney DVD called "Venice, Anyone?" which I played for her during our road trip to Venice. It was very hard to source a DVD player in 2017, but I managed to find one online.

As Mahra was still very small, all she needed for the trip was a couple of rattles and soft toys to keep her quiet. If you are able to travel while your children are under the age of one, I recommend it. It is easier than when they are toddlers.

Would They Eat the Food?

Shereena's favorite food during our European trip was penne pasta with white sauce. At every restaurant we went to, she would order either that or margarita pizza, which was not very hard for us to find. However, the year before, when we went to Ireland, her favorite food was rice and sour yogurt—a classic meal that a lot of children love to have here in the UAE. I loved this myself as a small child. So during our trip to Ireland, we only went to Indian and Lebanese restaurants that served white rice and yogurt, or to other restaurants that had white rice and we would bring in yogurt from a nearby grocery store.

Technology

I was completely against the use of iPads when my children were smaller. When Shereena was two, I decided to give her an iPad to enjoy during long drives to my parents in Sharjah or my husband's family in Al Ain. However, after just a few months I decided to ban the use of it. The main reason was that even though I'd installed a kids' YouTube app, weird videos would pop up that freaked the hell out of me. One showed a pregnant Elsa sitting on the bed with Batman doing pushups next to her. Now I don't know what message the creator of that video intended to convey to children, but I'm guessing it was nothing appropriate. Another one was of the "family finger" nursery rhyme that showed a hand with Donald Trump's and Hitler's heads as the fingers. Definitely disturbing! I did not want my children to be anywhere near such content! I finally decided to give Shereena an iPad when she started going to the "big girls' school." The school that I enrolled her at is Apple-certified, so a lot of the learning is based on the use of technology. I managed to install all educational apps and to ban YouTube. Kids are smart, though! I caught her one day typing "YouTube" into the browser! Luckily, I found a way to hide Safari from the iPad using the "restrictions" feature found in settings. At a later stage, I had to allow it back in so my daughter could access Education City, an educational resource that her school encouraged for home learning, but I found a way to allow access only to this website and nothing else.

I learned from this that sometimes as a parent, you have your own beliefs about what you want your child to see, especially when it comes to the use of technology, as the content displayed could have a huge impact on your child. But at some point, you might need to change your mind about your rules, so stay flexible.

And there you have it. All the real-life struggle I couldn't find in the books I bought and all the real-life messy truth that is part of being a Mom in the United Arab Emirates, as well as all the stories that I hope have shown you that you are going to be more than just okay—you are going to rock this parenting thing. It's not rocket science. It's not nuclear physics. It is hard and you will be tested as you never have before. But remember: you are mom, you do know best, and you can do this!